Biopsy Pathology
of the Endometrium

BIOPSY PATHOLOGY SERIES

General Editors

Professor Leonard S. Gottlieb, MD, MPH
Mallory Institute of Pathology,
Boston, USA

Professor A. Munro Neville, MD, PhD, MRC Path.
Ludwig Institute for Cancer Research,
Zurich, Switzerland

Professor F. Walker, MD, PhD, FRC Path.
Department of Pathology,
University of Aberdeen, UK

Biopsy Pathology of the Endometrium

C.H. BUCKLEY
MD, FRC Path

Senior Lecturer in Gynaecological Pathology, University of Manchester and Honorary Consultant Pathologist, St Mary's Hospital, Manchester

and

H. FOX
MD, FRC Path, FRCOG

Professor of Reproductive Pathology, University of Manchester and Honorary Consultant Pathologist, St Mary's Hospital, Manchester

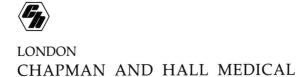

LONDON
CHAPMAN AND HALL MEDICAL

First published in 1989 by
Chapman and Hall Ltd
11 New Fetter Lane, London EC4P 4EE

© *1989, C.H. Buckley and H. Fox*

Typeset in 10/12pt Palatino by
EJS Chemical Composition, Bath
Printed in Great Britain at the
University Press, Cambridge

ISBN 0 412 23530 7

British Library Cataloguing in Publication Data

Buckley, C.H. (Cathryn Hilary)
  Biopsy pathology of the endometrium
  1. Women. Uterus. Endometrium.
  Histopathology
  I. Title II. Series III. Fox, H. (Harold)
  611'.018966

  ISBN 0 412 23530 7

Contents

Acknowledgements

We are deeply indebted to Linda Chawner for the invaluable help in the preparation of the illustrations. We are also grateful to Hazel Moore for the repetitive typing of our manuscript.

We are indebted to Richard Kempson of Stanford University for kindly supplying us with Figures 8.10 and 10.12 and to Robert Young of Harvard University for supplying us with Figure 12.3.

Preface

This volume is entitled *Biopsy Pathology of the Endometrium*. It is not intended to be a complete text on endometrial pathology and is strictly confined in content to the histological findings in endometrial tissue obtained by biopsy. We have chosen our illustrations from biopsy, rather than hysterectomy, specimens, as far as possible, achieving this aim in over 95% of the figures. Our only deviation from this rule has been in Chapter 2 in which we have utilized hysterectomy specimens to illustrate the morphological aspects of the endometrium during the normal menstrual cycle. Because, however, of our awareness that these cyclical changes, as seen in biopsy specimens, differ in many subtle ways from those apparent in intact uteri the changes described in Chapter 2 have to be contrasted with those discussed in Chapter 3, in which the cyclical endometrial changes, as seen in biopsy specimens, are considered.

Endometrial biopsies are often equated with 'curettings' and we have therefore interpreted our remit rather widely to include all specimens that may be received in the laboratory under this general heading. Thus, we have included chapters on abortion material and on gestational trophoblastic disease, neither of which should, in the strict sense, appear in a text on endometrial biopsies. In doing this, however, we have accepted the reality of the day-to-day situation in most histopathological laboratories, in which 'curettings' are grouped together as a single entity irrespective of whether they are truly endometrial biopsies or not.

We have attempted, throughout this volume, to stress the necessity for close co-operation between the pathologist and the gynaecologist. The gynaecologist must supply the pathologist with all the relevant clinical information required for an intelligent approach to the interpretation of endometrial biopsies. In return, the pathologist must extract from endometrial biopsies the maximum of information and convey this to the gynaecologist in clear terms.

C.H. Buckley
H. Fox

1 Sampling the endometrium

The term 'biopsy' is used to describe a tissue sample taken for pathological examination from the living person. Endometrial biopsy is undertaken to identify pathological processes within the endometrium, to obtain, indirectly, information about ovarian function and to assess the endometrial response to ovarian or exogenous hormones. The biopsy may be obtained from the endometrium by a curette without cervical dilatation, by aspiration, by endometrial wash or by endometrial brush as well as by cervical dilatation and curettage.

1.1 Techniques of endometrial sampling

1.1.1 Dilatation of the cervix with uterine curettage

The traditional method of removing endometrium for pathological examination is by dilating the cervix and methodically scraping tissue from the anterior and posterior walls of the uterine body with a curette. Many operators prefer to pass a pair of sponge forceps into the cavity prior to curettage as a means of identifying and removing polyps from within the cavity. Curettage provides an adequate, minimally traumatized, sample of endometrium which is generally easy to orientate and provides information about the functionalis and also, in many cases, about the basalis. It usually provides sufficient material for several techniques to be carried out on the same specimen, for example, microbiological examination, cryostat and routine paraffin processed sections and electron microscopy.

Curettage is most appropriate when a pathological process is suspected, for example for the diagnosis of hyperplasia or carcinoma, but, equally, provides an excellent sample for the assessment of the endometrial response to hormonal stimulation. In some cases, for example incomplete abortion, curettage is actually undertaken for therapeutic rather than diagnostic purposes; the resulting sample is, however, usually treated as a biopsy.

The technique may be refined in the investigation of neoplastic lesions by the process of fractional curettage, in which first the endocervical canal and then the uterine body are sampled in order to identify the origin of a tumour and determine the extent of its spread within the uterine cavity. Great care is required with this procedure if the samples are to represent accurately and separately the endometrium and endocervix without cross contamination.

The drawbacks to dilatation and curettage relate to the damage which may be inflicted on the cervix, during the dilatation, and the basalis, particularly when the endometrium is curetted in the postpartum period or when it is inflamed (see Asherman's syndrome). This technique is often considered to be unnecessarily traumatic for use during the investigation of infertility.

1.1.2   Single curettage

The taking of a single strip of the endometrium from the anterior or posterior uterine wall, without cervical dilatation, is a particularly suitable technique for the examination of the endometrium in patients with infertility. It causes minimal cervical and endometrial damage but allows, in the well-orientated sample, for an accurate assessment of the state of the endometrium as hormone-induced changes usually develop relatively uniformly throughout this tissue (Johannisson *et al*. 1982). It causes so little disturbance to the endometrium that repeat biopsy can be carried out in the same cycle. Single curettage is not suitable for the exclusion of pathological processes, their detection with this technique being often a matter purely of chance, particularly when the disease process is focal.

1.1.3   Aspiration, washes and endometrial brush techniques

Aspiration and endometrial wash techniques can be useful for the identification of a pathological process which may affect the entire endometrium and in which recognition of the abnormality does not depend upon the integrity of the tissue, but it is our personal experience that they are of very limited value for the interpretation of functional abnormalities.

The specimens tend to be small, are often fragmented (Figure 1.1) and may, therefore, be very difficult to orientate. They are, in some cases, more suitable for examination by cytopathological than histopathological techniques. They provide, however, a convenient out-patient procedure for the identification of gross endometrial pathology and are a moderately

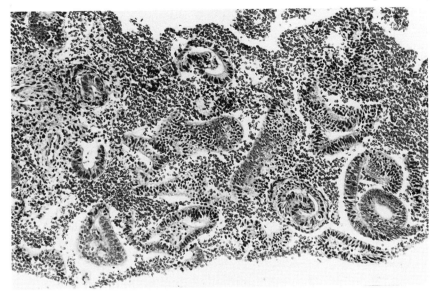

Figure 1.1   The fragmented tissue frequently seen in an aspiration biopsy. The inadequacy of this type of sample for detection of functional abnormalities is clearly apparent. Haematoxylin and Eosin × 186.

reliable means of correctly diagnosing carcinoma. It is unnecessary to carry out prior cervical dilatation and an anaesthetic is not required.

Endometrial brush samples are most appropriately examined by cytopathological techniques and are therefore outside the remit of this book.

1.2   Fixation of endometrial biopsies

In the majority of cases, only fixed, paraffin processed material will be examined and biopsies for this purpose should be placed in fixative as rapidly as possible after removal so as to prevent drying and autolysis. Of the fixatives in current use, Bouin's solution gives, in our view, the best results although there are many who prefer buffered formalin solution. A comparison between tissues prepared after fixation in the two fluids is illustrated in Figures 1.2 and 1.3.

Bouin's solution fixes small biopsies rapidly with excellent preservation of cell detail and tissues can be processed within two hours of their removal. It is, however, poorly penetrating and buffered formalin is preferred for larger pieces of tissue, such as bulky polyps. To the pathologist accustomed to interpreting formalin fixed tissue, it is

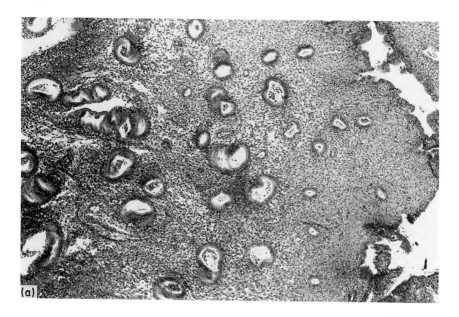

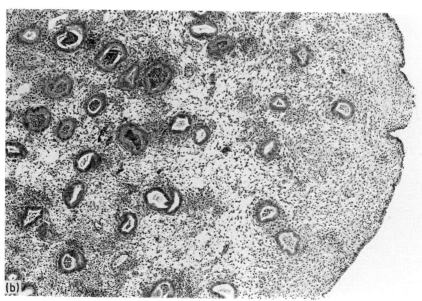

Figure 1.2 (a) Secretory endometrium with mild, active, non-specific, chronic inflammation, fixed in Bouin's fluid: biopsy from an IUCD user. Haematoxylin and Eosin × 47. **(b)** Part of the same tissue fixed in formalin. Haematoxylin and Eosin × 47. Glandular preservation is similar in the two samples but notice the apparent patchy distribution of the predecidua and the virtual absence of a compacta in the formalin fixed tissue, and the prominent compacta and extensive predecidualization in the Bouin's fixed sample.

4

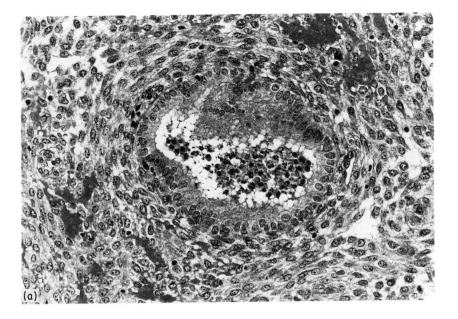

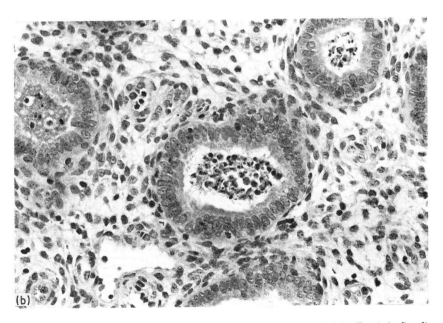

Figure 1.3 (a) A portion of the tissue shown in Figure 1.2 (a). (Bouin's fixed) Haematoxylin and Eosin × 232. **(b)** A portion of the tissue shown in Figure 1.2 (b). (Formalin fixed) Haematoxylin and Eosin × 232. Notice the better nuclear and cytoplasmic preservation, the ease with which the cellular detail can be identified and the presence of darkly staining intercellular stromal fluid in the specimen fixed in Bouin's solution.

necessary to adjust to the characteristic appearance of Bouin's fixed tissue in which the preservation of larger quantities of deeply staining inter-cellular fluid imparts an apparently increased density to the tissues. In the majority of cases Bouin's fixative does not hinder immuno-histochemistry and, in many instances, the more rapid fixation enhances the value of this technique.

Formalin fixes tissue relatively slowly and, as a consequence, tissues are less well preserved, mitoses more difficult to identify, nuclear chromatin patterns less clearly seen and interstitial fluids lost to a greater degree than in tissues fixed by Bouin's solution.

1.3   Processing and staining techniques

1.3.1   Paraffin processing

Most commonly endometrial biopsies are paraffin processed and sections, cut at 4 to 5 microns, are stained with haematoxylin and eosin. Some pathologists also like to examine a connective tissue stain, such as van Gieson, but it is not our practice to do so routinely.

P.A.S./Alcian blue stains, with and without prior digestion by diastase, are useful for the identification of glycogen, histiocytes (in inflammatory processes) and mucin in both neoplasms and metaplastic foci. Gram stains for bacilli, Ziehl-Neelsen stains for acid/alcohol fast bacilli and von Kossa stain for calcium are also useful in their place (see later). However, the range of stains used in the routine reporting of endometrial biopsies is very small.

1.3.2   Frozen sectioning

Frozen sections, stained with haematoxylin and eosin, may be carried out as a prelude to hysterectomy, when they are used to determine whether there is a non-neoplastic endometrial condition for which simple hysterectomy alone will suffice or if there is an endometrial neoplasm which necessitates hysterectomy and bilateral salpingo-oophorectomy with nodal dissection. The use of pre-hysterectomy frozen section has the advantage of obviating the need for two anaesthetics with their attendant morbidity. It should be appreciated, however, that many of the features by which we recognize the phases of the endometrial cycle in paraffin processed tissues are artifacts and that these will not be apparent in frozen material. A comparison between frozen material and the same specimen after Bouin's fixation and paraffin processing is shown in Figures 1.4 and 1.5. There are, however, a number of immunohisto-chemical techniques which require frozen rather than fixed tissues and

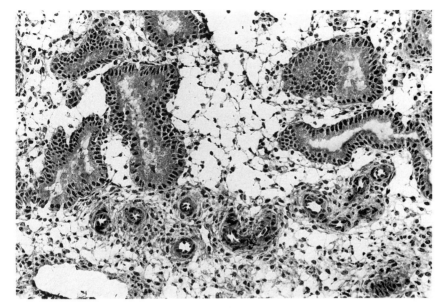

Figure 1.4 Cryostat section of a late secretory endometrium. Haematoxylin and Eosin × 186.

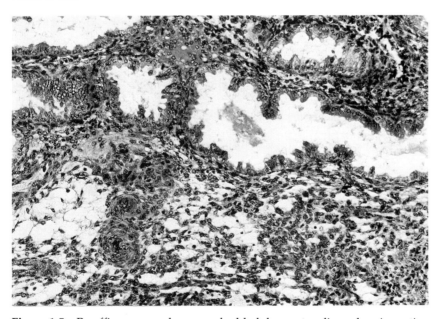

Figure 1.5 Paraffin processed, wax-embedded, haematoxylin and eosin section of the same tissue as that seen in Figure 1.4, × 186. Notice that the serrated configuration of the glands usually considered typical of the late secretory phase is absent from the frozen material but that the spiral arteries and their surrounding cuff of predecidua are similar in the two sections.

many monoclonal antibodies will give satisfactory results only on frozen material.

1.3.3 Electron microscopy

It has been our experience that electron microscopy is seldom required in the diagnosis of routine endometrial samples. Its use appears to be limited to the recognition of the occasional poorly-differentiated neoplasm and even here its contribution is minimal; in general more useful information is obtained from the judicious and more economical use of immunohistochemical techniques. It is not proposed, therefore, to describe the electron-optic appearances of the normal endometrium or the pathological processes which affect it because it is our belief that knowledge of these will seldom be required.

1.3.4 Immunohistochemistry

Immunohistochemical examination of the endometrium is undertaken most frequently for the identification of neoplastic conditions. Both frozen material and paraffin processed tissue are suitable for this purpose. The techniques are adequately described in standard texts on the subject (Polak and Van Noorden, 1986) and will not be discussed in detail here.

1.4 Timing and siting of endometrial biopsies

In order to obtain the maximum information from an endometrial biopsy it is important for the clinician first to provide accurate and complete clinical details and secondly for the sample to be taken at the optimum time and from the appropriate site in the uterus. The request form should, at least, provide the date of the last menstrual period and, preferably, the date of ovulation or basal temperature change, together with information concerning the use of any steroid hormones, mode of contraception, use of any drugs known to interfere with the normal secretion of trophic hormones, details of any endocrinological disease, and such aspects of the past medical history as are required to explain the need for the examination. The menstrual history is essential and should be insisted upon.

1.4.1 Site of the endometrial biopsy

Endometrial biopsies should be taken from the anterior or posterior wall in the uterine body where cyclical changes are likely to be most adequately developed. The tissue of the uterine isthmus fails to undergo cyclical changes and a common error of the inexperienced surgeon is to sample the endometrium too low down in the cavity. Basal endometrium also fails to show normal cyclical changes and therefore the immediately postmenstrual biopsy may fail to provide useful information.

In addition to operator errors, there are naturally occurring phenomena which may result in the removal of an unrepresentative sample. For example, the endometrium overlying a submucous leiomyoma is frequently shallow, may contain fewer than normal glands and in extreme cases may be represented by only a single layer of columnar epithelium with a little underlying stroma (Figure 1.6). The tissue in this area may also be ulcerated or focally inflamed. In the patient wearing an IUCD, removal of tissue only from the contact site may give a false impression of infection, irregular ripening or scarring.

1.4.2   Timing of the endometrial biopsy

It may be impossible, in the presence of endometrial lesions which produce abnormal bleeding, to select accurately the time at which to take the biopsy but this may have little adverse effect on the detection of those

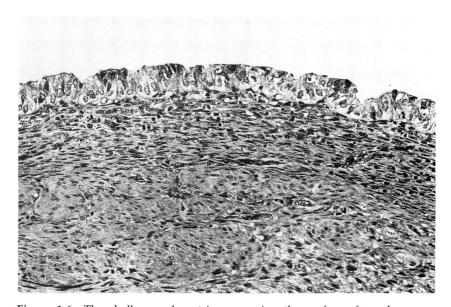

Figure 1.6   The shallow endometrium covering the surface of a submucous leiomyoma. Glands are absent and the surface epithelium is separated from the myometrium by only a wisp of endometrial stroma. Haematoxylin and Eosin × 232.

pathological processes which may be identified at any time, whether the patient is actively bleeding or not, for example the hyperplasias and neoplasms. In fact, if a pathological process is suspected there is little to gain and a great deal to lose by postponing the biopsy and, indeed, waiting for the bleeding to cease may result in complete loss of the abnormal endometrium and thus hinder diagnosis (Dallenbach-Hellweg, 1987). However, the appearances of cyclical hormone-related conditions and inflammatory processes vary according to the stage of the cycle and careful timing of such biopsies is required.

The best time for observing cyclical changes in the endometrium is between the 7th and 11th post-ovulatory days. At this stage it is possible to assess both the adequacy of the secretory change and its uniformity. It should also be possible to identify an inflammatory process if one is present, although tuberculosis may be difficult or impossible to recognize until the 12th or 13th post-ovulatory day.

In the two days prior to menstruation, inflammatory changes, with the exception of tuberculosis, are difficult to identify with certainty in haematoxylin and eosin stained sections because they are masked by the physiological stromal cellular infiltrate which accompanies the late secretory phase. This is, however, the optimum time for identifying tuberculosis but as acid/alcohol fast bacilli are notoriously difficult to identify in endometrium and, as morphologically well-developed tubercles are an unusual finding, it is essential for simultaneous microbiological studies to be carried out.

The sample which to the histopathologist is the most difficult to interpret, and hence the least satisfactory, is the menstrual sample. It may only be possible, at best, to determine whether bleeding has occurred from a secretory endometrium, and is therefore actually menstrual, or whether bleeding is the result of hormonal withdrawal in a non-secretory endometrium. Its most useful purpose is for microbiological studies.

References

Dallenbach-Hellweg, G. (1987) Functional disturbances of the endometrium. In *Haines and Taylor: Obstetrical and Gynaecological Pathology* (ed. H. Fox), Churchill Livingstone, Edinburgh, pp. 320–39.

Johannisson, E., Parker, R.A., Landgren, B.M. and Diczfalusy, C. (1982) Morphometric analysis of the human endometrium in relation of peripheral hormone levels. *Fertil. Steril.*, **38**, 564–71.

Polak, J.M. and Van Noorden, S. (1986) *Immunocytochemistry: Modern Methods and Applications*, 2nd edn, Wright, Bristol.

2 The anatomy and histology of the endometrium

The uterine cavity is approximately triangular in coronal section with the apex below at the internal os and the base of the triangle at the fundus of the uterus. In sagittal section it is slit-like because the anterior and posterior walls are almost in contact (Gray, 1980). The length of the cavity varies, measuring up to 5.0 cm in the reproductive years and often less than 2.0 cm in the postmenopausal years.

2.1 The normal endometrium

The endometrium forms the lining of the uterine body from the isthmus below to the commencement above of the interstitial segments of the Fallopian tubes in the uterine cornua, on each side of the fundus. It is characterized by its striking sensitivity to ovarian hormones, its lability and its remarkable regenerative capacity. It undergoes regular cyclical changes, in response to the recurrent hormonal changes of the ovulatory cycle, during the reproductive years and provides a dormant mucous membrane for the uterus prior to the menarche and after the menopause.

The endometrium is composed of simple, tubular glands set in a cellular, vascular stroma (Figure 2.1). There are two components, a basal layer, or basalis, which does not respond to hormonal stimulation under normal circumstances, and a more superficial layer, the functionalis, which responds to the hormonal changes of the normal ovulatory cycle and is regularly shed and regenerated during the reproductive years. There is no sharp line of demarcation between the functionalis and basalis and the junction between the basal endometrium and myometrium is rather irregular and ill-defined (Figures 2.2 and 2.20). The depth of the functionalis varies throughout the menstrual cycle, reaching its maximum in the late proliferative or mid-secretory phase and being shallowest in the immediate postmenstrual phase; it is absent in the premenarchal and postmenopausal states.

In the uterine cornua there is a transition to tubal mucosa which may be

11

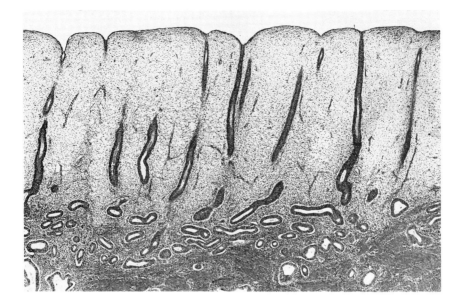

Figure 2.1 Early proliferative phase endometrium, 8th day of cycle. Straight, narrow tubular glands are set in a fragile immature cellular stroma in which there are only thin-walled blood vessels. The stroma of the basalis is more densely cellular than that of the functionalis but there is no sharp line of demarcation between these two zones or between the basalis and underlying myometrium. Haematoxylin and Eosin × 30.

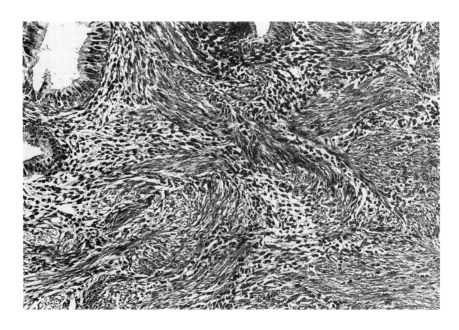

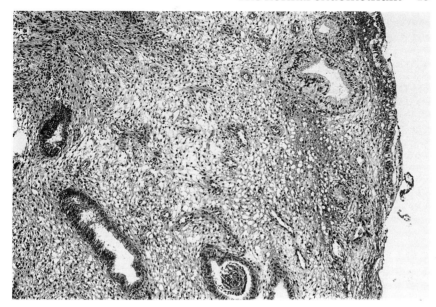

Figure 2.3   The uterine isthmus. Glands lined by epithelium of endometrial type lie to the left and the crypts, to the right, are lined by mucus-secreting epithelium of endocervical type. Mucus-secreting epithelium also covers the surface of the tissue; the stroma is more fibrous than in the uterine body. Haematoxylin and Eosin × 93.

abrupt or gradual and in a proportion of women endometrium extends for some way into the interstitial segments of the Fallopian tubes.

In the uterine isthmus, the cellular endometrial stroma is gradually replaced by a less cellular, more fibrous, connective tissue resembling that of the cervix and epithelium of both endometrial and endocervical type is seen (Figure 2.3).

2.1.1   Basal endometrium

The stroma in basal endometrium is more densely cellular than in the functionalis and nucleocytoplasmic ratios are high: thus, on microscopic

Figure 2.2   The ill-defined junction between the basalis and the myometrium. The smaller, randomly distributed, more darkly staining cells of the endometrial stroma are seen in the upper part of the field and the myometrium with interweaving bundles of large, elongated smooth muscle cells with copious pale cytoplasm lie below. Haematoxylin and Eosin × 186.

examination, the tissue is generally basophilic. A scattering of lymphocytes and lymphoid aggregates is common and constitutes part of the
normal structure; thick-walled arteries are present (Figures 2.4 and 2.5).
At its deep border the basalis blends with the myometrium and there is a
narrow zone in which endometrial stromal cells and smooth muscle are
intermingled (Figure 2.2).

The glands are often less evenly distributed in the basalis than in the
functional layers (Figure 2.4) and are mildly irregular. They are lined by
a columnar epithelium with tall, closely packed narrow cells with
elongated, parallel-sided, or rather cigar-shaped, nuclei orientated at
right angles to the basement membrane (Figure 3.6); a minor degree of
pseudostratification may be seen. The appearances of the basalis are more
or less constant throughout the normal cycle.

2.1.2   Isthmic endometrium

In the upper part of the isthmus the stroma is similar to that in the body
but it becomes progressively more fibrous, less cellular and more
eosinophilic, in haematoxylin and eosin stained sections, as the

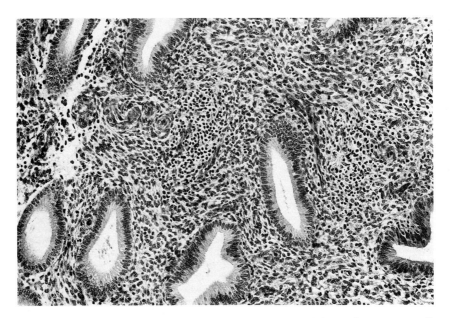

Figure 2.4   Basal endometrium. The stroma is densely cellular and contains small
lymphoid aggregates; these are normally seen in the basalis. The glands are
narrow and lined by a tall columnar epithelium. Haematoxylin and Eosin × 186.

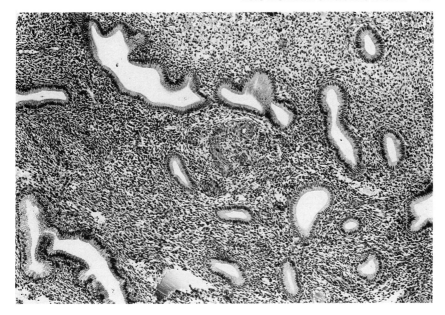

Figure 2.5 Basal endometrium. The basal glands are more irregularly dispersed and more variable in size and shape than in the functionalis. Thick-walled muscular arteries, which do not vary throughout the cycle, are seen in the centre of the field. Haematoxylin and Eosin × 93.

proportion of collagen gradually increases so that in the lower isthmus it comes to resemble the fibrous stroma of the endocervix: thin-walled venous and capillary channels are present and, depending on whether it is upper or lower isthmus, the surface epithelium is of endometrial or endocervical type respectively (Figure 2.3). In the isthmus, the glands are more widely spaced than in the true endometrium, are often a little dilated and are lined by epithelium of endometrial type which is either unresponsive to normal hormonal stimulation or lags behind that of the body (Figure 2.6) (Hendrickson and Kempson, 1980).

2.1.3   Functional endometrium

The functionalis is the superficial layer of the endometrium which normally develops only during the reproductive years, its structure and activity accurately reflecting the pattern of ovarian hormone secretion. It may also grow under the influence of abnormal endogenous or exogenous oestrogens (Chapter 5). During the reproductive cycle, the functionalis undergoes regular growth and maturation which terminate, in the absence of pregnancy, in its being shed, on average, every 28 days.

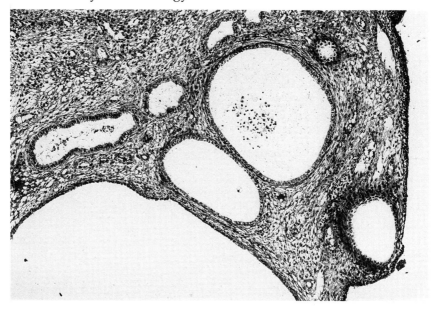

Figure 2.6   The uterine isthmus. The glands, which are lined by epithelium of endometrial type, are cystically dilated and there is no evidence of cyclical changes. Haematoxylin and Eosin × 93.

It is customary, in the United Kingdom, to speak of the reproductive cycle as commencing on the first day of menstruation, though in some countries the day of ovulation is regarded as the start of the cycle. It is of course much easier to be certain of the date of the last menstrual period than of the date of ovulation, except in those uncommon patients in whom hormone levels are being monitored.

The cyclical changes in the functionalis may be described either in terms of the predominant endometrial morphological features or, alternatively, in terms of the ovarian cyclical hormone secretion. Thus we speak of the proliferative or follicular phase of the cycle, corresponding to the phase of ovarian follicular growth prior to ovulation, and of the secretory or luteal (post-ovulatory) phase after ovulation has occurred. In the normal cycle, the post-ovulatory phase is remarkably constant, lasting 14 days, and variations in cycle length are usually due to alterations in the follicular or proliferative phase of the cycle which may vary from 8 to 21 days.

During the phase of ovarian follicular growth, in response to pituitary follicle stimulating hormone, oestradiol, the most potent of the ovarian oestrogens, and oestrone, a weaker and less important oestrogen, are secreted by the granulosa and thecal cells of the developing follicle.

Secretion reaches a peak just before ovulation, declines briefly in the early post-ovulatory phase and then increases again, to a rather lesser extent, due to oestrogen secretion by the corpus luteum, finally falling to resting levels in the immediate premenstrual phase as the corpus luteum degenerates. During the initial phase of follicular growth oestrogen is responsible for the co-ordinated growth of the endometrial glands, stroma and vasculature and for the induction of progesterone receptors and, during the second, minor peak, for the oedema which characterizes the mid secretory phase.

Following ovulation, the ovarian follicle develops into the mature corpus luteum and this coincides with a rapid rise in progesterone secretion, although the first detectable increase occurs in response to the mid-cycle luteinizing hormone (LH) surge which immediately precedes ovulation. Progesterone levels reach a peak 3 to 4 days after ovulation, but are usually sufficient to induce changes in the endometrium within 24 to 36 hours of ovulation. They remain high until 2 or 3 days before the end of the cycle, and then, in the absence of pregnancy and as the corpus luteum degenerates, decline rapidly. Progesterone is responsible for the development in the endometrium of the glandular secretory changes which become apparent 24 to 36 hours after ovulation, for stromal maturation or decidualization and for differentiation of the spiral arteries which proceeds throughout the post-ovulatory phase.

2.1.4   The phases of the endometrial cycle

During the proliferative phase of the cycle, the appearances of the endometrium do not differ sufficiently from day to day for the precise stage of the cycle to be identified but following ovulation the changes in the secretory endometrium are so specific that it is possible to identify the duration of the phase to within 1 or 2 days (Noyes *et al.* 1950). As a consequence, even when precise dating of the endometrium is not required, it is usual to describe the secretory endometrium in terms of its major morphological changes as being in the early, mid or late secretory phase.

(a) *Postmenstrual   and   proliferative   (follicular   phase)*   Immediately following menstruation, which lasts on average 5 days, the uterus is lined only by basal endometrium and the residuum of the deeper part of the functionalis. Regrowth commences, even in the absence of hormonal stimulation, on the 3rd to 4th day and is first evidenced by a healing of the surface epithelium (Figure 2.7). Subsequently, between the 5th and 14th days of the 'typical' 28-day cycle, the proliferative or follicular phase, there is synchronous stromal, glandular and vascular growth, the

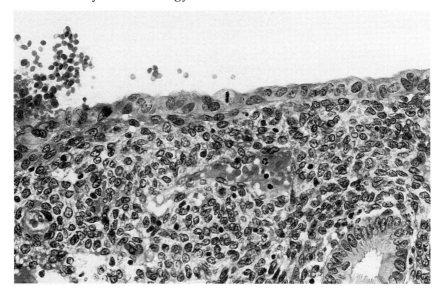

Figure 2.7   Basal endometrium in the late menstrual phase (4th day of the cycle). Regeneration of the surface epithelium is characterized by focal immaturity, loss of cellular polarity, mild pleomorphism and the presence of mitotic figures. Haematoxylin and Eosin × 370.

endometrium increasing in depth until the time of ovulation, the 14th day of the cycle.

In the early part of the proliferative phase the glands are straight and tubular and the stroma immature (Figure 2.1). Later in the phase, from day 10, glandular growth outstrips that of the stroma; the glands thus become progressively more convoluted (Figure 2.8) and mild stromal oedema may develop.

(b)   *Secretory phase*   The secretory phase is characterized by glandular secretion and stromal maturation, these occurring in response to progesterone produced by the corpus luteum. These changes occur only when progesterone receptors are present in the endometrium and the development of these, in turn, depends upon there having been adequate oestrogen secretion in the follicular phase, progesterone receptors being oestrogen-induced.

The secretory phase is divided into three stages, the early secretory phase lasting from the 2nd to 4th post-ovulatory day, the mid secretory phase extending from the 5th to 9th post-ovulatory day and the late secretory phase from the 10th to 14th post-ovulatory day.

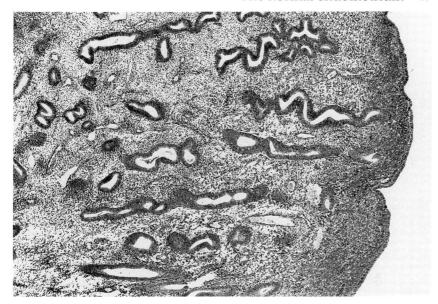

Figure 2.8   Late proliferative phase endometrium, 12th day of cycle. The glands remain simple tubular and parallel-sided but are rather tortuous and mildly convoluted. There is slight stromal oedema. Haematoxylin and Eosin × 47.

Secretion is not apparent in the glands until 24 to 36 hours after ovulation, this being sometimes known as the interval phase. After the interval, in response to the rising progesterone levels, first, secretory changes become apparent in the glandular epithelium and, later, predecidual changes occur in the stroma.

Early secretory phase: The glandular morphology of the early secretory phase is similar to that of the late proliferative phase and the first presumptive evidence of ovulation is the appearance, in the glandular epithelium, of subnuclear vacuoles (Figures 2.9 and 3.13). These normally appear on the 16th day of the cycle (2nd post-ovulatory day). They are initially few in number and irregularly distributed throughout the sample but within 12 hours they become more uniform and can be detected in most glands; they reach a peak between the 17th and 18th day of the cycle (3rd and 4th post-ovulatory day), the early secretory phase (Figures 2.10 and 3.15). It can be assumed that ovulation has occurred only when vacuoles are uniformly distributed in at least 50% of the glands.

Mid secretory phase: Between the 19th and 23rd days of the cycle (5th to 9th post-ovulatory day), the mid secretory phase, secretion of the glandular epithelial contents occurs, reaching a peak on the 21st day (7th

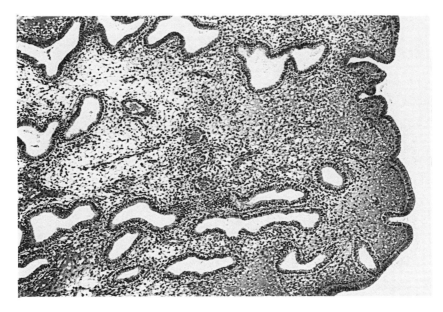

Figure 2.9 Endometrium in transition from proliferative to early secretory phase (2nd to 3rd post-ovulatory day). The glands retain the rather tortuous appearance of the late proliferative phase (Figure 2.8) but there are vacuoles in the infranuclear cytoplasm of some of the cells in the glandular epithelium. Haematoxylin and Eosin × 93.

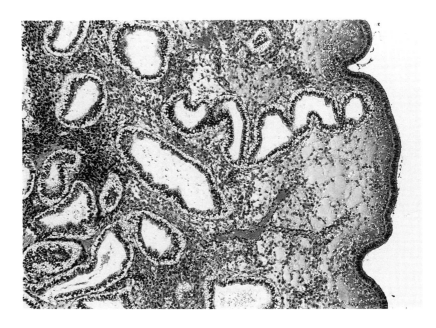

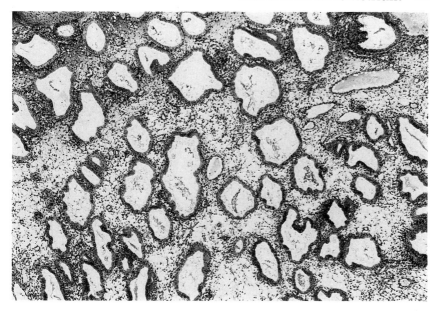

Figure 2.11 Mid-secretory endometrium, 7th to 8th post-ovulatory day. Glandular secretion has reached a peak, the lumina are distended and the glands appear somewhat angulated in cross section. Stromal oedema is marked and spiral arteries are inconspicuous. Haematoxylin and Eosin × 60.

post-ovulatory day), and it is at this stage of the cycle that the most satisfactory biopsy for the assessment of secretory activity is obtained (Figures 2.11 and 3.16). Stromal oedema, which is first apparent in the early secretory phase, reaches a peak on days 22 to 23 and by day 23 spiral artery differentiation is apparent, becoming more obvious on day 24 (Figure 2.12). The vessels proliferate, pericytes widen, myofibrils differentiate and at the same time perivascular stromal cells become more conspicuous, their cytoplasm increasing in quantity and eosinophilia; these predecidual cells first become apparent on day 23 (9th post-ovulatory day).

Late secretory phase: The late secretory phase (days 24 to 28, 10th to 14th post-ovulatory day) is characterized by exhaustion of glandular secretory

Figure 2.10 Early secretory endometrium, 4th post-ovulatory day. Prominent subnuclear vacuoles are uniformly distributed throughout the glandular epithelium and the stroma is mildly oedematous. A minor degree of glandular luminal distension is now apparent. Haematoxylin and Eosin × 93.

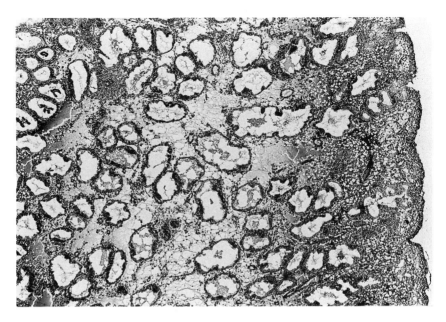

Figure 2.12 Endometrium in transition from mid to late secretory phase, 10th post-ovulatory day. Secretion is past its peak and minor glandular serrations are apparent. Stromal oedema is still prominent and spiral arteries are visible, each with a narrow cuff of predecidua. Haematoxylin and Eosin × 47.

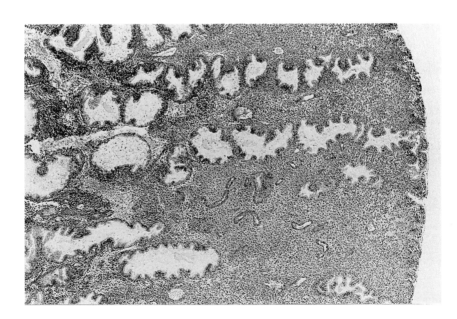

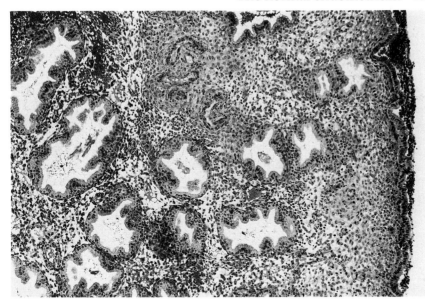

Figure 2.14 Late secretory endometrium, 13th to 14th post-ovulatory day. The glandular outline is so markedly serrated that the epithelium appears tufted where tangential cutting has occurred. A cuff of predecidua surrounds the spiral artery, which is well muscularized and tortuous, and a compact layer has differentiated. Haematoxylin and Eosin × 93.

activity, the glands become serrated and tortuous, and there is a general reduction in endometrial height due to regression of the stromal oedema (Figures 2.13 and 3.18). Predecidual change develops in the stromal cells which form a cuff around the spiral arteries and a compact layer below the surface epithelium (Figures 2.14, 3.17 and 3.19). Apart from the cuff of predecidua around the spiral arteries, the stroma in the mid zone of the functionalis shows little predecidual change and hence appears less opaque or solid on histological examination; this is the spongy layer. A stromal infiltrate composed predominantly of K-cells, but also containing the occasional polymorphonuclear leucocytic cluster, characterizes the immediate premenstrual stroma (Figure 3.21). K-cells or 'endometrial

---

Figure 2.13 Late secretory endometrium, 12th post-ovulatory day. Glandular secretion is exhausted and stromal oedema has been lost; as a consequence, the glands have collapsed and appear serrated. A wide cuff of decidualized cells surrounds the spiral arteries, which are well muscularized, and a band of predecidua lies immediately deep to the surface epithelium. Haematoxylin and Eosin × 47.

granulocytes' have a lymphocyte-like nucleus and a variable number of phloxinophilic cytoplasmic granules. The origin and function of these cells has been much debated but it is now clear that they are granulated lymphocytes (Bulmer *et al.*, 1987) and it is possible that they play a role in the immunological interaction between maternal and fetal tissues.

(c)   *Menstrual phase*   Evidence of the onset of menstruation is apparent by the 28th day of the cycle, before the patient has noticed any bleeding (Figure 2.15). Over the next 24 hours a plane of separation becomes apparent (Figure 2.16) through the spongy layer, which leads to the separation of the superficial endometrium (Figure 2.17) from the basal, a variable amount of functional endometrium remaining attached to the basalis (Figure 2.18).

2.1.5   *Postmenopausal endometrium*

As ovulation ceases at the time of the menopause and oestrogen secretion diminishes, endometrial growth is no longer stimulated though the precise appearance of the endometrium is somewhat variable.

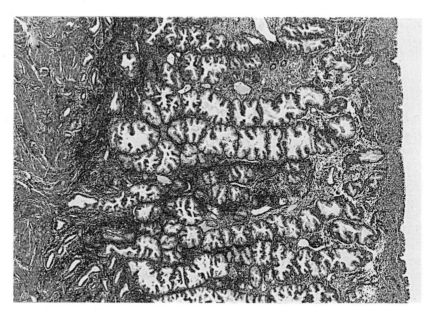

Figure 2.15   Early menstrual endometrium, first day of the cycle. Glandular serration is greatly exaggerated in comparison with that which is seen in Figure 2.13, approximately 24 hours earlier in the cycle. There is disruption of the stroma immediately deep to the compacta with aggregation of stromal cells and interstitial haemorrhage. Haematoxylin and Eosin × 37.

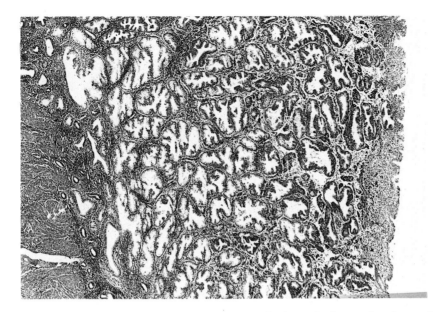

Figure 2.16 Menstrual endometrium, second day of the cycle. Stromal aggregation is more pronounced, disruption of the stromal skeleton has occurred, and there is separation of the glands and stroma. Haematoxylin and Eosin × 30.

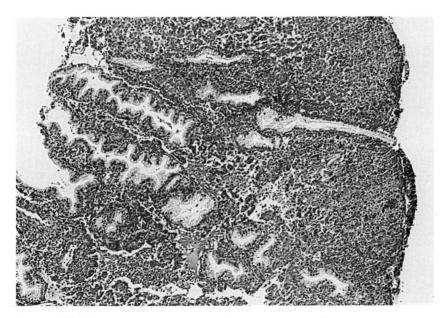

Figure 2.17 Menstrual endometrium. Fragments of superficial endometrium as they appear shed in a curettage sample taken on the first day of bleeding. Haematoxylin and Eosin × 93.

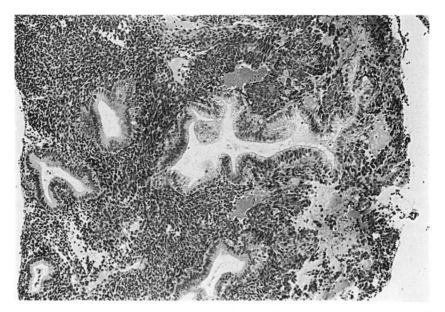

Figure 2.18 Menstrual endometrium, 4th day of the cycle. The compacta and underlying spongy layer have been shed and the uterus is lined only by basal and residual secretory endometrium; the ragged endometrial surface is seen to the right. Haematoxylin and Eosin × 117.

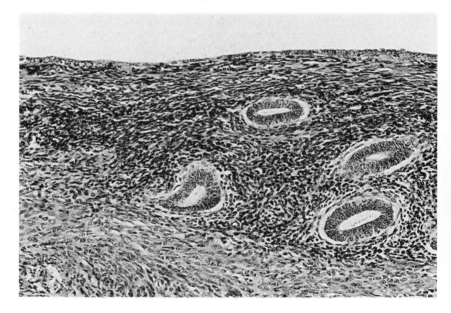

Figure 2.19 Postmenopausal endometrium. The uterus is lined by a shallow endometrium with compact stroma and scanty tubular glands lined by epithelium exhibiting mild stratification and having scanty cytoplasm. Haematoxylin and Eosin × 186.

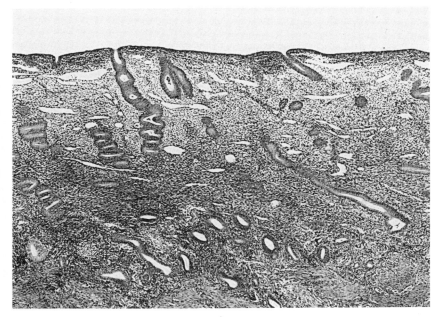

Figure 2.20 Postmenopausal endometrium. The uterus is linked by an inactive endometrium but a shallow, relatively translucent functional layer is seen. Note the irregularity of the endometrial/myometrial junction and the blending of the basal and functional layers. Haematoxylin and Eosin × 47.

In the absence of oestrogen there is no functionalis and the uterus is lined only by a shallow basalis (Figure 2.19), similar in appearance to that seen in the reproductive years. The stroma is cellular and the small, narrow, tubular glands are lined by a cuboidal epithelium of indeterminate type. The line of demarcation between the myometrium and endometrium often becomes more coarsely irregular than in the reproductive years and it may be difficult to distinguish endometrial stroma from myometrium (Figure 2.20). Several years after the menopause the stroma may have become fibrous and the typical stromal cellularity diminished.

Alternatively, and often some years after the menopause, the endometrial glands may become cystically dilated and lined by a single layer of flattened cuboidal epithelium of indeterminate type: the stroma is often partially or sometimes predominantly fibrous (Figure 2.21). This is the picture of so-called senile cystic atrophy and it is not unusual for the cystic areas to become somewhat polypoidal. The cystic dilatation of the atrophic glands is probably a result of blockage of the gland necks by fibrous tissue. This appearance has, in the past, often been classed as a form of postmenopausal hyperplasia but the atrophic inactive

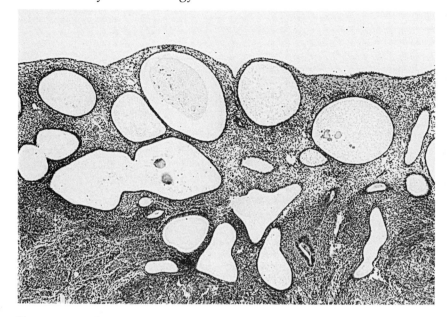

Figure 2.21 Postmenopausal endometrium, senile cystic change. The endometrium is shallow and the stroma compact but the glands, even those in the basalis, are cystically dilated. Haematoxylin and Eosin × 60.

appearance convincingly negates any concept of a proliferative process. It is also of note that the incidence of cystic change in the endometrium is highest in women who are many years past their menopause and lowest in those whose menopause was in the relatively recent past: this clearly indicates that senile cystic atrophy is not, as has frequently been claimed, a residuum of a regressed perimenopausal endometrial hyperplasia.

If, following the menopause, reduction of oestrogen occurs to a lesser degree, or more slowly, the endometrial glands may be lined by a mildly pseudostratified columnar epithelium in which mitoses may be seen for some time (up to 2 years) after the clinical menopause (Figure 2.20). In such cases a shallow layer of functionalis can also be seen as a very thin, superficial layer of less densely cellular stroma in which straight tubular glands are present: mitoses are not seen in the stroma.

References

Bulmer, J.N., Hollings, D. and Ritson, A. (1987) Immunocytochemical evidence that endometrial stromal granulocytes are granulated lymphocytes. *J. Pathol.,* **153**, 281–7.

Gray's Anatomy (1980) 36th edn. (eds P.L. Williams and R. Warwick), Churchill Livingstone, Edinburgh, pp. 798 and 1428–31.

Hendrickson, M.R. and Kempson, R.L. (1980) *Surgical Pathology of the Uterine Corpus*, W.B. Saunders, Philadelphia, London, Toronto.

Noyes, R.N., Hertig, A.T. and Rock, J. (1950) Dating the endometrial biopsy. *Fertil Steril.*, **1**, 3–11.

3   The normal endometrium as seen in biopsy material

Endometrial samples from normal women in the reproductive years vary in their content according to the mode of sampling and, often, according to the purpose for which they are intended. The size and adequacy of the sample therefore depends not so much upon the quantity of endometrium present in the body of the uterus as on clinical practices and we would regard it as unwise to draw any conclusions about endometrial volume from a biopsy specimen.

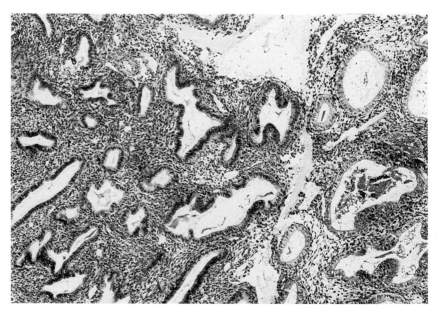

Figure 3.1 Basal and functional endometrium as they appear in a curettage sample. To the left, the basal glands are somewhat irregular, lined by a darkly staining, inactive columnar epithelium and set in a compact cellular stroma. On the right, the functional glands are in transition from early to mid secretory phase, are rather dilated and the stroma is less compact. Haematoxylin and Eosin × 93.

The quality of the sample will also vary according to the type of fixative used and the time interval between removal of the specimen and its placing in fixative (Chapter 1). These are factors over which the pathologist may have limited control but which must, of necessity, be taken into account when interpreting endometrial biopsies.

The tissues in an endometrial biopsy are rarely ideally orientated and each individual component must be recognized and its significance evaluated if false conclusions about the variability of the endometrial appearance and maturation are to be avoided.

It is usual to find both functional and basal endometrium in curettage samples (Figure 3.1) whilst, in some cases, particularly in the postabortive or postpartum state when the tissues are soft, myometrium may be encountered (Figure 3.2). Fragments of endocervical and ectocervical tissue are also commonly present (Figure 3.3). In biopsies which have been taken from infertile patients simply in order to assess the quality of secretory change and exclude overt disease, it is usual to expect only functionalis and aspiration samples are usually small and fragmented, even to the extent that epithelial and stromal fragments lie separately (Figure 1.1).

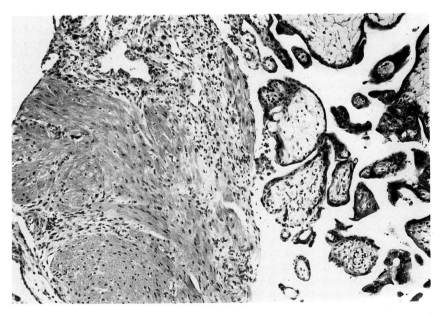

Figure 3.2 Myometrium in a curettage specimen. Smooth muscle and basal endometrium lie to the left and placental villi to the right. From a patient who suffered a spontaneous abortion. Haematoxylin and Eosin × 117.

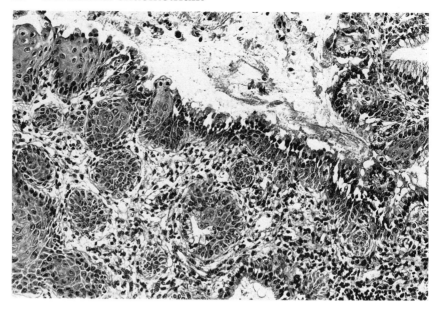

Figure 3.3   Endocervical tissue in which the surface and crypt epithelium has undergone squamous metaplasia; such fragments are common in endometrial curettings and usually come from the lower part of the endocervical canal. Care should be taken to distinguish the mucus-secreting epithelium of the cervix from the superficially similar secretory epithelium of the endometrium. Haematoxylin and Eosin × 186.

3.1   The isthmus

Isthmic tissue may be included intentionally in the biopsy as part of a single endometrial strip taken to sample the entire endometrium from the fundus to the isthmus and in these cases it is clearly recognizable, the transition from endometrium to isthmus being easy to identify (Figure 3.4). Isthmic tissue may also be intermingled with fragments from the body or cervix and care must be taken to recognize these lest they convey the wrong impression to the pathologist (Figure 3.5).

Tissue from the isthmus differs from that in the body in so far as the stroma contains a higher proportion of fibrous tissue whilst glands with characteristics of both the endometrium and endocervix are seen. A well-taken and well-orientated sample should present no difficulties in recognition but, in practice, irregularly orientated material is most commonly seen. It is important to remember, particularly when isthmic tissue forms the major component of the sample, that the isthmic glands and stroma do not mirror the hormonal-dependent changes in the uterine

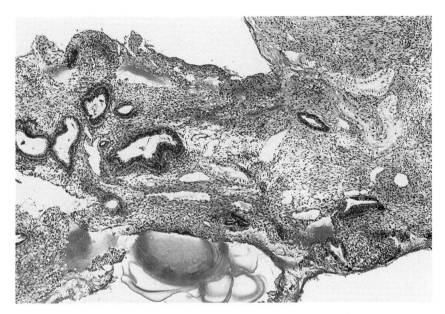

Figure 3.4 A strip of endometrium taken to include the isthmus. The upper end of the tissue, in which there are glands of endometrial type, lies to the left and endocervical crypts are seen on the right. Haematoxylin and Eosin × 60.

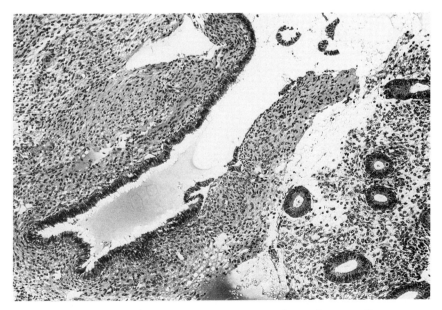

Figure 3.5 Isthmic tissue and proliferative endometrium as they appear intermingled in a curettage sample. Haematoxylin and Eosin × 117.

body and are thus unsuitable for determining the quality of such changes (Figure 2.6).

3.2   Basal endometrium

It is usual to see fragments of basal endometrium in curettage samples but not in the more superficial biopsies taken in the investigation of infertility or obtained by an aspiration technique. Basal tissues are easy to identify when they are orientated in their correct anatomical position in relation to the functionalis. Difficulties are sometimes encountered, however, when fragments of basalis are received mixed with functionalis, when basalis is cut in transverse section or when curettage has taken place shortly following an episode of bleeding, this having left basalis as the only endometrium available for sampling. In this last case, it is particularly important to recognize that the tissue is basalis or the pathologist may reach the erroneous conclusion that the endometrium is inactive.

The appearance of the basalis remains constant throughout the normal cycle (Figure 3.6). The stroma is densely cellular, the individual spindled

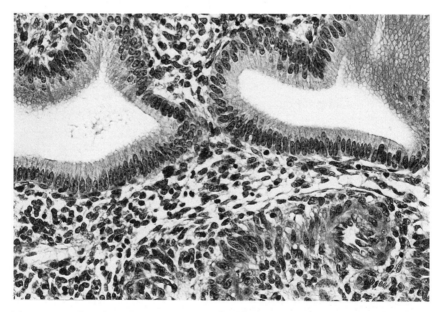

Figure 3.6 Basal endometrium. The glands are lined by a tall, columnar epithelium, which in the reproductive years has pale cytoplasm, parallel-sided, closely packed nuclei and low nucleo-cytoplasmic ratios. Contrast this with the cells lining the glands in the postmenopausal patient (Figure 3.22). The thick-walled artery is typical of the basalis. Haematoxylin and Eosin × 370.

cells having oval to elongated darkly staining nuclei, scanty cytoplasm and ill-defined cell borders. The glandular epithelium in the basalis is columnar. The cells appear tightly packed, have more scanty cytoplasm than in the functionalis and are orientated at right angles to the basement membrane of the gland, their nuclei being tall and strikingly parallel-sided. Mitoses are not seen.

3.3 Menstrual phase

Biopsies taken during menstruation are often difficult to interpret and provide very limited information. They are composed largely of blood in which collapsed, serrated glands, aggregates of stromal cells and small clusters of neutrophilic polymorphonuclear leucocytes are intermingled (Figure 3.7). The normal morphology is lost after the first day of menstruation and, apart from confirming that the material came from a secretory endometrium and is thus actually menstrual and that bleeding

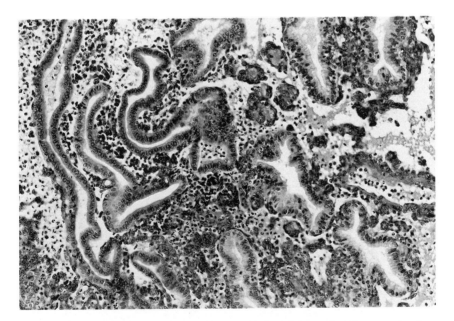

Figure 3.7   Menstrual endometrium, second day of the cycle. The sample often consists of no more than isolated glandular elements intermingled with stromal cell aggregates and blood clot. Secretory activity can usually still be identified in the glandular epithelium confirming that this is in fact menstrual and not oestrogen or therapeutic hormone withdrawal bleeding (see Figure 5.16). Haematoxylin and Eosin × 186.

is not the consequence of oestrogen withdrawal, the pathologist may be unable to supply any further information.

On the first day of the cycle (Figure 3.8), in vertically orientated tissue continuous segments of serrated, collapsed glands, including their orifices, lie in a haemorrhagic, fragmented stroma in which the stromal cells form densely cellular clusters and are admixed with neutrophil polymorphonuclear leucocytes. Aggregation of the stromal cells and interstitial haemorrhage, indicative of the onset of menstruation, are identifiable first in the spongy layer of the functionalis (Figure 2.15), and it is at this level that the plane of cleavage will occur. The decidual appearance of the stromal cells, so characteristic of the late secretory phase, is lost as the stromal cells aggregate, although K-cells are still apparent. Spiral artery remnants also remain identifiable. The glandular epithelium is usually described as being exhausted but in practice, even at this stage, the epithelium in some glands, particularly around the margin of the sample where fixation occurred most rapidly, remains vacuolated and of secretory appearance (Figure 3.9). In horizontally orientated material stellate glandular remnants are seen in a fragmented stroma.

By the second to third day of the cycle little or no stromal tissue may

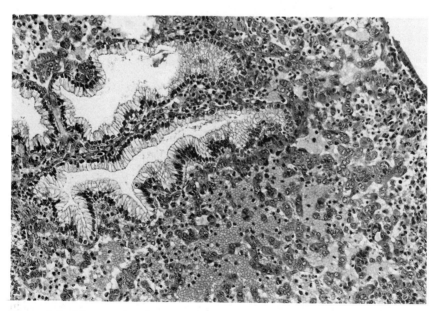

Figure 3.8   Menstrual endometrium, first day of the cycle. Secretory glands are set in a haemorrhagic stroma in which the cells have undergone aggregation. Haematoxylin and Eosin × 186.

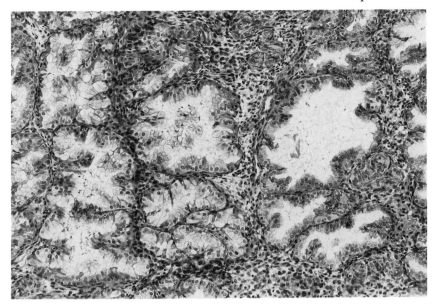

Figure 3.9 Menstrual endometrium, first day of the cycle. The cells lining the glands to the left of the tissue are large, have prominent round nuclei and more copious cytoplasm than in the glands to the right. This 'pseudo-hypersecretory' appearance is a fixation artifact. The glands showing this phenomenon lie closer to the surface of the tissue and therefore become more rapidly fixed. Haematoxylin and Eosin × 149.

remain and the glands, which appear more resistant to dissolution than the stroma, become closely packed (Figure 3.7) and are seen in the biopsy in a virtually back-to-back pattern. They may therefore bear a superficial resemblance to a hyperplastic endometrium or even to an adeno-carcinoma. Careful attention to the cytological details should clarify the position.

By the 3rd to 4th day of the cycle, towards the end of the menstrual phase, the functionalis has been largely lost, only tiny dense basophilic cellular aggregates of indeterminate type remaining (Figure 3.10). A biopsy taken at this stage now often contains basal endometrium and the adjacent residual functionalis in which there are the remnants of secretory glands (Figure 2.18). The surface is ragged and fragmented and there is no epithelial covering but healing of the surface epithelium, from the glandular epithelium, is apparent by the 3rd to 4th day (Figure 2.7). This process appears to be independent of hormonal stimulation and therefore mitoses are often seen here even when they are absent in the

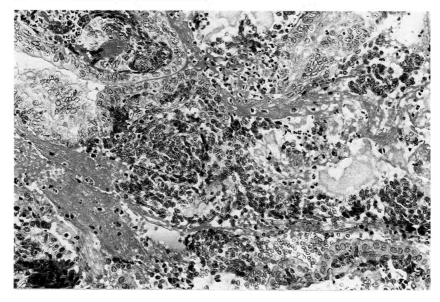

Figure 3.10   Menstrual endometrium, 3rd day of the cycle. The sample consists only of blood clot containing stromal cellular aggregates, isolated epithelial fragments and blood. Haematoxylin and Eosin × 232.

deeper parts of the glands. No abnormal mitoses occur but the epithelial cells often show a minor degree of reactive cytological atypia during healing.

3.4   Proliferative (follicular) phase

It is impossible precisely to date the endometrium in the proliferative phase but in an adequate sample some idea of the duration and adequacy of the phase can be gained from the depth of the functional layer, the degree of glandular development and tortuosity and the number of stromal and epithelial mitoses.

In the early part of the proliferative phase (days 5 to 7), the glands are straight, narrow (Figure 2.1) and round in cross section (Figure 3.11); their moderately basophilic epithelium is cubo-columnar with oval or rounded nuclei in which the chromatin is evenly dispersed. There is a minor degree of epithelial stratification. Occasional mitoses are seen in the glandular epithelium and are identified most easily, at this stage, in that part of the glands lying in the junctional zone between the basalis and functionalis; they may therefore be scanty in a superficial biopsy. The

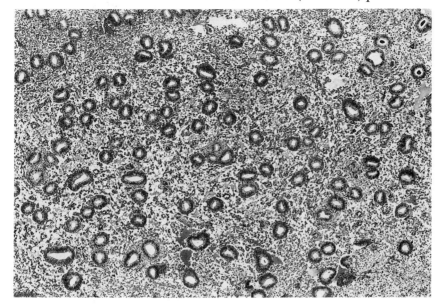

Figure 3.11   Proliferative phase endometrium. A transverse section through the narrow, tubular glands emphasizes their uniformity of shape and distribution. Haematoxylin and Eosin × 37.

stromal cells show mitotic activity and are oval to elongated with scanty cytoplasm and ill-defined cell borders; the delicate, translucent appearances of the newly grown functional stroma is in sharp contrast to the darkly staining, dense, underlying basalis. Scanty thin-walled blood vessels are present and the fibrous endometrial skeleton is identifiable.

Proliferative activity reaches its maximum between the 8th and 10th days of the cycle and by then the glandular epithelium is taller, stratification of the epithelium is more obvious and mitotic figures are frequently seen in both the glands and stroma (Figure 3.12). Transient mild stromal oedema is common and capillaries are numerous although arteries and arterioles are inconspicuous.

In the late proliferative phase (days 11 to 14), glandular growth outstrips that of the stroma and, as a consequence, the glands become rather tortuous. They therefore appear in section as more variable in size and shape (Figure 2.8), but it is helpful to remember that their walls remain parallel no matter how oblique the plane of section. The glandular epithelium remains stratified but mitoses decline in number in both the glands and stroma.

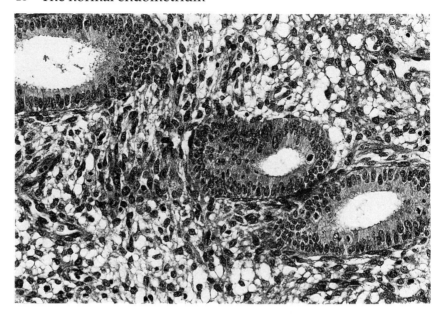

Figure 3.12 Mid-proliferative phase endometrium, 9th to 10th day of the cycle. Glandular epithelium is pseudostratified and the nuclei oval or elongated; stromal cells are immature and cell membranes and cytoplasm ill-defined. Mitoses are visible in both the glandular and stromal cells. Haematoxylin and Eosin × 297.

3.5 Secretory phase

In contrast to the proliferative phase, the appearances of the endometrium in the secretory phase can be fairly precisely related to the day of the cycle. As the investigation of infertility becomes more sophisticated, with parallel sequential hormone measurements, it is useful to advise the gynaecologist as to the number of days since ovulation when reporting a secretory phase endometrium.

3.5.1 Early and mid secretory phase

Following ovulation there may be no change in the appearance of the endometrium for between 24 and 36 hours but at the end of that time vacuoles appear in the subnuclear cytoplasm of the glandular epithelium (Figure 3.13). In the first 12 hours these are somewhat irregularly dispersed, being most marked in the parts of the glands in the mid zone of the endometrium and least obvious in the superficial part, and occurring in some but not all the cells in a particular gland. The presence of the vacuoles appears to exaggerate the stratification of the nuclei. Not until

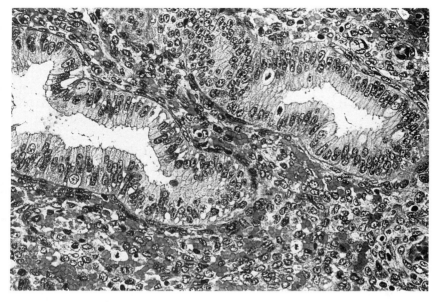

Figure 3.13 Endometrium in transition from proliferative to early secretory phase, second post-ovulatory day. The glands retain the tubular form and pseudostratified epithelium characteristic of the proliferative phase but scanty subnuclear vacuoles are present in the glandular epithelium. Haematoxylin and Eosin × 370.

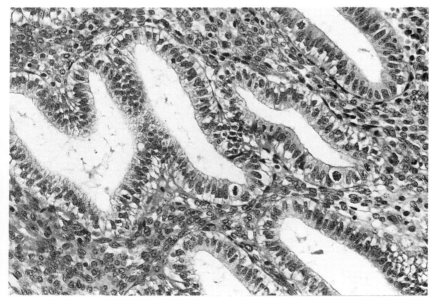

Figure 3.14 Early secretory endometrium, 3rd post-ovulatory day. Although mitoses are still present in the glandular epithelium, subnuclear vacuoles are now uniformly distributed. Contrast with Figure 3.13. Haematoxylin and Eosin × 297.

the vacuoles are evenly distributed in at least 50% of the glands can one be certain that ovulation has occurred (early secretory phase). At this stage mitoses are still common in the glandular epithelium; in fact they will be identified in small numbers until the 17th day (Figure 3.14). Gland profiles remain similar to those of the proliferative phase until day 18 when subnuclear vacuoles reach their peak (Figure 3.15) but, with the movement of the vacuolar contents from the subnuclear cytoplasm to the supranuclear cytoplasm and then into the glandular lumina, there is a progressive distension of the glands which reaches a peak on day 21 to 22 (the 7th to 8th post-ovulatory day), i.e. during the mid secretory phase. This creates the typical geometrical shape of the mid secretory gland (Figure 3.16) which develops as secretions distend a gland tethered by the supporting stroma. As secretion of cell contents occurs the nuclei return to a basal position in the cells and careful examination of the cell tips reveals a shaggy appearance. Secretion is usually fairly uniform throughout the specimen but the glands tend to be a little narrower and less actively secretory in the superficial functionalis, the part that will eventually develop into the compacta of the late secretory phase (Figure 3.17). Biopsies that include only this part of the endometrium may

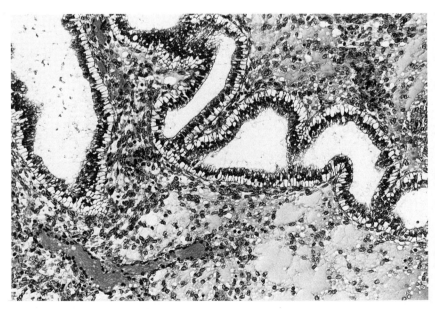

Figure 3.15 Early secretory phase endometrium, 4th post-ovulatory day. Subnuclear vacuolation of the glandular epithelium is uniform and at its peak and stromal oedema is present. Haematoxylin and Eosin × 186.

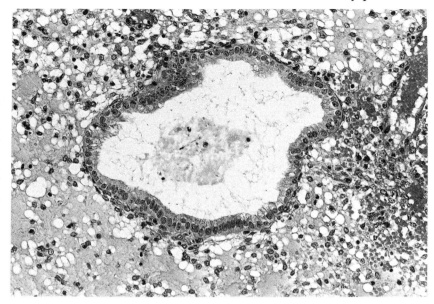

Figure 3.16 Mid secretory endometrium, 8th post-ovulatory day. The gland is rather angular in outline, is distended and contains a trace of secretion. The glandular epithelium is tall, the regular oval nuclei have returned to the base of the cells and the surrounding stroma is markedly oedematous. Haematoxylin and Eosin × 232.

therefore give a false impression of poorly developed, narrow, weakly secretory glands.

The stroma of the early secretory phase (post-ovulatory days 1 to 5) differs very little from that typical of the follicular phase but towards the end of the early secretory phase there is a progressive accumulation of oedema fluid in the stroma which reaches a peak in the mid secretory phase on the 22nd to 23rd day of the cycle (8th to 9th post-ovulatory day) (Figure 2.11). Stromal oedema is maximal in the spongy layer, in the mid zone of the endometrium, and this will persist to some extent into the late secretory phase. The amount of oedema fluid which is apparent in paraffin processed material depends upon the fixative (Chapter 1) and it is important that one should become familiar with the normal appearances which occur using the different fixatives.

3.5.2   *The late secretory phase*

In the late secretory phase glandular secretion is exhausted, the glands collapse, their lumina become narrow, particularly in the most superficial

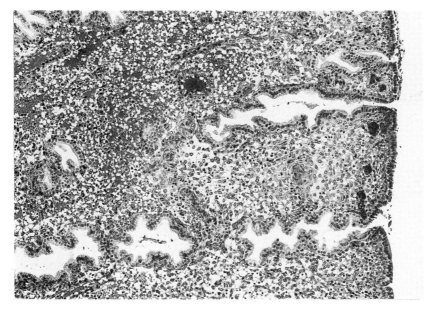

Figure 3.17 Late secretory endometrium, 12th post-ovulatory day. The superficial segments of the glands as they pass through the compacta are rather narrow and a biopsy in which the tissue is orientated so that the plane of section passes through these narrower segments may give a false impression that glandular development is inadequate. Haematoxylin and Eosin × 117.

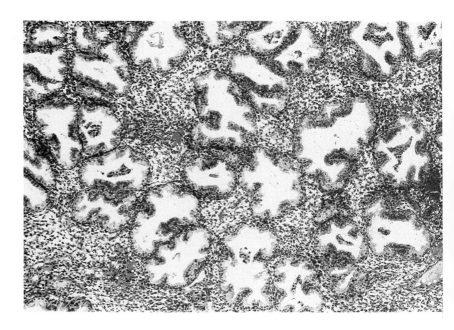

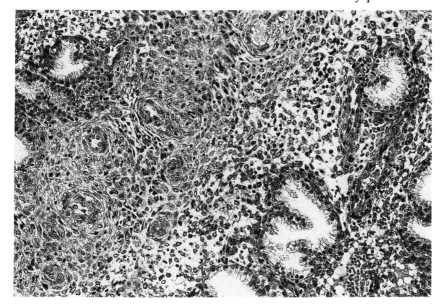

Figure 3.19 Late secretory endometrium, 13th post-ovulatory day. The spiral artery to the left is well-muscularized and surrounded by a cuff of pre-decidualized stromal cells with regular round nuclei, copious cytoplasm and well-defined cell margins. Haematoxylin and Eosin × 93.

part of the gland (Figure 3.17), and their contour becomes saw-toothed (Figure 2.15). Associated with the reduction in endometrial height, which results from the regression of stromal oedema, the glands become plicated (Figure 3.18).

Spiral artery growth occurs throughout the proliferative phase but maturation of the muscular layer only becomes evident at the end of the mid secretory phase on day 22 (8th post-ovulatory day). Stromal predecidualization occurs first in the mid-zone of the endometrium, around the spiral arteries, on the 23rd day (9th post-ovulatory day). It increases rapidly over the next two days appearing in the infraluminal stroma on day 25. By the end of the cycle a distinct, superficial, compact layer has formed and bands of predecidua traverse the spongy layer along the course of the spiral arteries (Figure 3.19).

Figure 3.18 Late secretory phase endometrium, 13th post-ovulatory day. Loss of oedema in the spongy layer has resulted in close packing of the glands which are now well past the secretory peak and have become irregular and rather serrated. Haematoxylin and Eosin × 93.

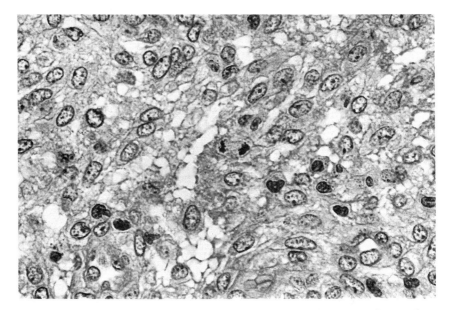

Figure 3.20 Late secretory endometrium, 13th to 14th post-ovulatory day. Within the compacta there is a sparse infiltrate of darkly staining granulated lymphocytes (K-cells) and a mitosis is seen in a stromal cell. Haematoxylin and Eosin × 743.

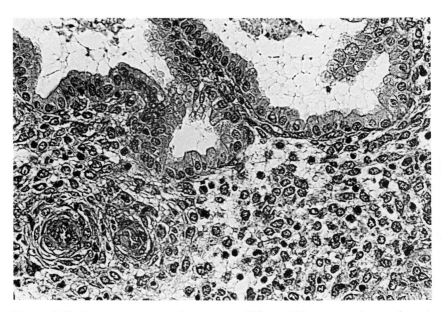

Figure 3.21 Late secretory endometrium, 13th to 14th post-ovulatory day. A scattering of granulated lymphocytes is present in the stroma and two, well-muscularized spiral arteries are seen on the left. Haematoxylin and Eosin × 370.

Mitoses reappear in the stroma by day 26 or 27 (Figure 3.20) and are a reflection of the decrease in progestagenic activity which allows a minor recrudescence of an oestrogenic effect. On days 27 and 28 granulated lymphocytes (K-cells) appear (Figure 3.21) and a scattering of neutrophil polymorphs infiltrates the superficial stroma in the immediate premenstrual phase.

3.6   Postmenopausal endometrium

In the postmenopausal woman, the endometrium is shallow and endometrial biopsy samples are therefore often scanty if not actually inadequate. Frequently the material consists only of isolated fragments of inactive cubo-columnar epithelium of indeterminate type and fragments of fibrous stroma. In these circumstances it may be possible only to tell the gynaecologist that there is no evidence of neoplasm or proliferative activity but quite impossible to comment upon any other characteristics of the tissue.

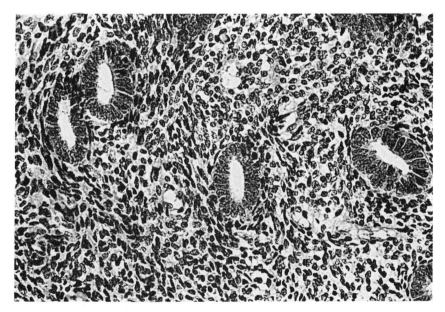

Figure 3.22   Postmenopausal endometrium, the last menstrual period had occurred 10 months previously. The stroma is composed of closely packed cells with scanty cytoplasm; the glands are narrow, tubular and lined by a single layer of cubo-columnar cells with very little cytoplasm. Contrast with the appearance of the basal glands in the reproductive years (Figure 3.6). Haematoxylin and Eosin × 370.

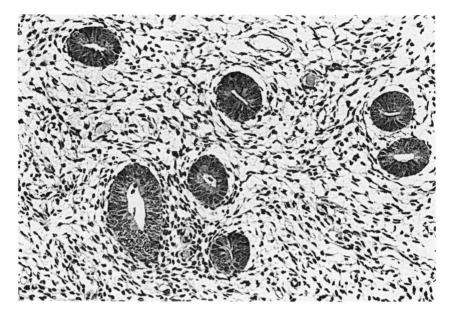

Figure 3.23 Weakly proliferative, postmenopausal endometrium. The glandular epithelium is mildly stratified and the stroma less compact than in the sample shown in Figure 3.22. Haematoxylin and Eosin × 232.

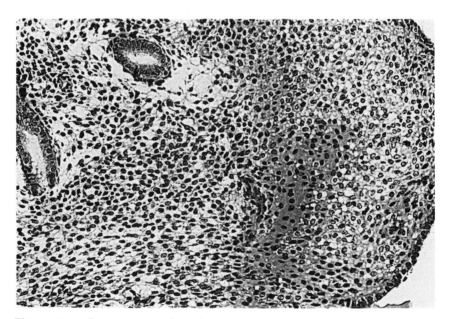

Figure 3.24 Postmenopausal endometrium in which continued, low-level oestrogen stimulation has resulted in the formation of a shallow functionalis recognized by the less compact stroma and the resemblance of the cells to those seen in the proliferative phase (Figure 3.12). Haematoxylin and Eosin × 232.

In a more adequate sample, narrow tubular glands lined by cuboidal epithelium showing neither secretory nor proliferative activity (Figure 3.22) are set in a compact cellular stroma. The epithelium may remain tall and, on occasions, mildly pseudostratified (Figure 3.23) and a shallow functionalis may persist for many years after the menopause. This is indicative of the presence of persistent very low levels of oestrogen of either endogenous or exogenous origin, e.g. from topical oestrogens used to treat vaginal atrophy (Figure 3.24). Glandular mitoses are also sometimes encountered in patients in whom there is no proven source of oestrogenic stimulation but in whom there is a genital prolapse. More commonly the picture of very weak proliferative activity is seen in women who have experienced postmenopausal bleeding in the years immediately following the menopause or in women in whom the menopause appears to be occurring gradually over a period of years.

Many years after the menopause, the stroma may become fibrous and this is a particularly conspicuous feature in women developing senile cystic atrophy (Figure 3.25). The glands vary in size, some being narrow and tubular but many are dilated and cystic. The glandular epithelium is

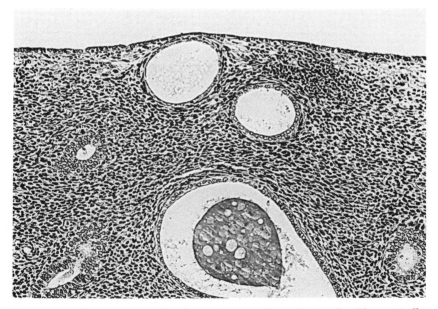

Figure 3.25 Postmenopausal endometrium, senile cystic atrophy. The cystically dilated glands are lined by a single layer of inactive, flattened cubo-columnar cells. Compare this with the tall stratified columnar epithelium lining the glands in simple hyperplasia (Figure 9.1). Haematoxylin and Eosin × 186.

inactive and cuboidal but in the most widely dilated glands it may be flattened and of indeterminate type. Such endometrium has a tendency to become polypoidal and this may be apparent in the biopsy.

It is also noticeable that in the postmenopausal phase there may be an increase in the number of lymphocytes and the number of lymphoid aggregates, these features appearing to occur without evidence of overt infection. The development of lymphoid follicles with germinal centres, however, is normally regarded by us as indicating the development of infection.

4 Functional disorders of the endometrium

Those abnormalities of endometrial development and maturation which are secondary to ovarian dysfunction are usually referred to as functional disorders. This term encompasses endometrial abnormalities due to a paucity of oestrogen, an excess of oestrogen, an abnormality of progesterone secretion following ovulation or an abnormality in the relative proportions of oestrogen and progesterone.

4.1 Endometrial atrophy and low or absent oestrogen states

An atrophic endometrium and low oestrogen state are typical of the normal pre-menarchal child and of the postmenopausal woman (Chapter 3) but occur under pathological conditions in the absence of normal ovarian follicular development, following irradiation damage to the ovaries and in primary or secondary ovarian failure. Endometrial atrophy is therefore encountered in women with a wide range of abnormalities, some of which may be ovarian, e.g. 17-hydroxylase deficiency, gonadotrophin-resistant ovary syndrome, premature menopause, whilst others lie in the hypothalamic-pituitary axis, e.g. hypopituitary states, hyperprolactinaemia.

Patients with abnormally low oestrogen levels may present with delayed puberty, delayed menarche, primary amenorrhoea, oligo-menorrhoea or infertility, the clinical picture depending upon the patient's age and the severity of the abnormality. The appearance of the endometrium is, however, similar in all instances whatever the nature of the primary abnormality as it simply reflects the inadequacy of oestrogenic stimulation. A similar picture is seen in those uncommon patients in whom ovulatory function is normal but in whom the endometrium is refractory to hormonal stimulation (Dallenbach-Hellweg, 1987).

The degree of endometrial atrophy varies, but in cases of the most profound oestrogen deficiency it is complete, the uterus being lined only by endometrium of basal type (Figure 2.19). There is no functionalis and

51

biopsy samples tend to be scanty and rather difficult to obtain. Biopsy of the endometrium reveals an inactive picture (Figure 3.22). The stroma is composed of closely packed, spindle-shaped cells and appears densely cellular; the glands, which are usually sparse, simple and tubular, are lined by an inactive, cuboidal or cubo-columnar epithelium with scanty cytoplasm and densely staining nuclei. In women in whom oestrogen levels are lower than the physiological range, but are nevertheless sufficient to induce a minimum of growth, there can be a minor degree of glandular epithelial stratification, occasional mitoses may be seen and a thin functionalis can form (Figure 4.1).

In patients with inadequate, rather than absent, follicular function a paucity of oestrogen in the follicular phase may lead to prolongation of the proliferative phase without the development of a hyperplastic endometrium. In such patients biopsy may reveal a morphologically normal endometrium which is delayed relative to the apparent day of the cycle or a weakly proliferative endometrium. Some patients in this category will, in due course, if oestrogen secretion is not opposed by a progestagen, develop a mild complex hyperplasia, the so-called

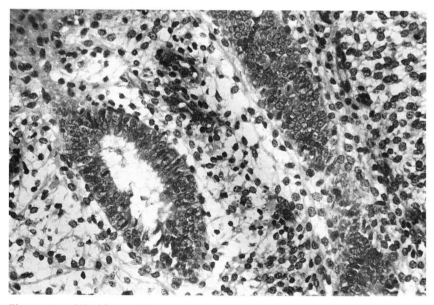

Figure 4.1 Weakly proliferative endometrium in a low oestrogen state. The glands are lined by a mildly stratified epithelium in which occasional mitoses are seen. The stroma is immature. Only scanty curettage material was received. Haematoxylin and Eosin × 370.

disordered proliferative endometrium (Chapter 7). Inadequate oestrogen secretion is also a factor in the development of luteal phase insufficiency (see below).

4.2   Anovulatory cycles and hyperoestrogenic states

The term 'hyperoestrogenic state' implies that the endometrium is being subjected to unopposed oestrogenic stimulation. Oestrogen levels are therefore not necessarily elevated, for normal levels of oestrogen, the action of which is not opposed or interrupted by progesterone, can produce a hyperoestrogenic state as is the case, for instance, in women having anovulatory cycles. A genuine hyperoestrogenic state with abnormally high oestrogen levels is rather uncommon but is seen, for example, in women with the polycystic ovary syndrome or with granulosa cell tumours of the ovary. It is the case, of course, that true hyperoestrogenism of this type will also result in anovulatory cycles by disturbing the hypothalamic feedback mechanism. Clinically the patient

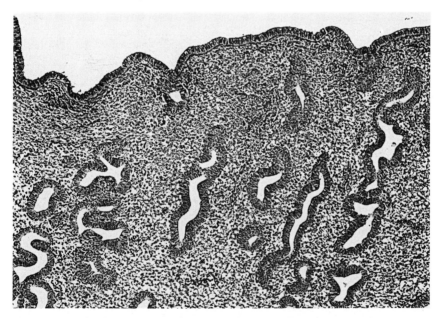

Figure 4.2 Prolonged proliferative phase endometrium. The patient menstruated only every 45 to 50 days; the last menstrual period had occurred 34 days previously. The endometrial glands are not dissimilar from those seen in the normal late proliferative phase but are slightly more tortuous; there is no evidence of hyperplasia. Haematoxylin and Eosin × 93.

may have oligomenorrhoea, amenorrhoea, infrequent heavy vaginal bleeding interspersed with episodes of scanty vaginal loss, infertility or any combination or permutation of these problems.

Persistent or prolonged stimulation of the endometrium by oestrogens, uninterrupted by progestagenic activity, results ultimately in the development of an endometrial hyperplasia of simple or atypical form. The appearances are similar whatever the source of the oestrogen and are fully described in Chapter 7.

In some patients, however, the changes are insufficient to warrant a diagnosis of hyperplasia but are recognizable as those of a prolonged proliferative phase (Figures 4.2 and 4.3). Mitotic activity continues beyond the 14th day of the cycle, glandular epithelial stratification persists, a minor degree of variation in glandular size is seen, without gross cystic dilatation, a little focal glandular crowding can be present and the stroma remains immature and cellular. These features occur in women in whom there is a failure or delay of ovulation in the current cycle, for example due to a persistent, unruptured follicle, or in whom there has been a previous anovulatory cycle. A prolonged proliferative phase may be followed by either a normal or an inadequate luteal phase (see below).

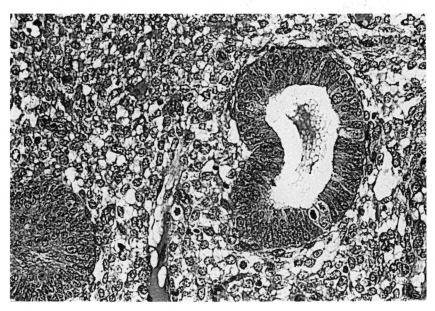

Figure 4.3 Prolonged proliferative phase endometrium. There is mild stratification of the glandular epithelium; mitoses are present in both glands and stroma. Haematoxylin and Eosin × 370.

4.2.1   Oestrogen withdrawal bleeding

Bleeding from an endometrium subjected only to oestrogenic stimulation (oestrogen withdrawal bleeding) can be recognized in endometrial biopsies. In hypo-oestrogenic states curetting typically yields a scanty sample in which inactive glands, showing no evidence of secretory activity, are admixed with fragments of both crumbling and intact haemorrhagic endometrium. A history of surprisingly severe or prolonged bleeding may be obtained which seems to be at variance with the paucity of the sample. There is frequently a scanty to moderately heavy endometrial stromal infiltrate of lymphocytes, macrophages (some of which may contain haemosiderin) and plasma cells, this feature being seen particularly in the woman who has had repeated or prolonged bleeding.

Bleeding after, or during, a hyperoestrogenic state is characteristically irregular. The endometrium is bulky and biopsy usually yields pieces of relatively well-preserved endometrium in which areas showing focal interstitial haemorrhage and stromal disintegration are interspersed with intact proliferative or inactive endometrium showing little or no evidence of interstitial haemorrhage. A scattering of polymorphonuclear leucocytes is commonly found in the areas of stromal disintegration (Figure 9.3).

4.3   Luteal phase insufficiency

The terms 'luteal phase insufficiency' and 'secretory insufficiency or inadequacy' are used to describe a state characterized by a relative or absolute abnormality in progesterone secretion following ovulation. This abnormality probably occurs sporadically in normal women but in those in whom it is thought to be the cause of clinical symptoms the diagnosis should be confirmed by repeated biopsies over several cycles.

An inadequate luteal phase can be preceded by a normal, short or inadequate follicular phase. Following ovulation, there may be a delay in progesterone secretion, a general paucity of progesterone secretion with a failure to reach physiological levels, a gradual rather than rapid rise in progesterone secretion, a premature decline in progesterone levels towards the end of the phase (short secretory phase), abnormal persistence of an active corpus luteum beyond fourteen days or a relative deficiency of progesterone associated with hyperoestrogenism. The condition is most accurately expressed in terms of the hormonal abnormality but there are a number of morphological features which may alert the histopathologist to this diagnosis.

56   Functional disorders

Patients with luteal phase insufficiency may have apparently normal menstrual cycles, but many complain of premenstrual spotting, a blood-stained vaginal discharge for several days prior to the onset of menstruation, intermenstrual bleeding, irregular cycles, prolonged, though not necessarily heavy, periods or infertility. The histopathological features do not always correlate directly with either the hormone levels or the clinical symptoms, although some pictures are sufficiently specific as to suggest the nature of the underlying hormonal abnormality. Others simply allow the pathologist to suggest the possible nature of the underlying problem. The biopsies vary greatly in appearance and several patterns are recognizable.

4.3.1   Co-ordinated delayed endometrial transformation

In its simplest form, the endometrium is of normal morphology but shows a co-ordinated delay in glandular and stromal maturation relative to the day of ovulation. Such a picture may occur when progesterone

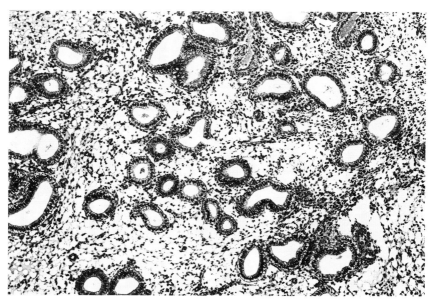

Figure 4.4 Luteal phase insufficiency, 8th post-ovulatory day. Subnuclear vacuoles are still present in the epithelium of the majority of glands and the stroma is immature, an appearance corresponding approximately to the 3rd post-ovulatory day. Little glandular dilatation has occurred. Occasional less mature glands are also seen indicating a minor degree of irregular ripening. Haematoxylin and Eosin × 93.

secretion following ovulation is delayed, or the rise in progesterone levels is slow or inadequate. In such cases it may be impossible to recognize the abnormality unless the gynaecologist has given the date of ovulation (Figure 4.4). In other cases, however, if the inadequate luteal phase follows a prolonged follicular phase the endometrium may show secretory changes superimposed upon an endometrium which exhibits features of a prolonged follicular phase (see above), an underlying simple hyperplasia or, less commonly, an atypical hyperplasia. Biopsies of this type may be seen in patients with an apparently normal menstrual cycle but the biopsy may show not only delay in maturation but also, frequently, premature breakdown (see below).

4.3.2   Generally inadequate secretory phase, glandular stromal asynchrony and irregular ripening

In patients with luteal phase insufficiency preceded by, or associated with, oestrogen deficiency the endometrium is poorly grown and shallow and the biopsy may be scanty and include basal endometrium or myometrium (de Brux, 1981a). The glands are sparse, straight, narrow

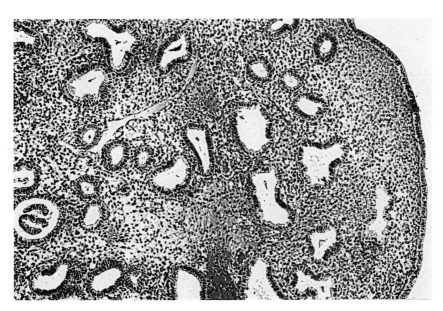

Figure 4.5 Luteal phase insufficiency. The endometrium is poorly grown, most glands are narrow and are devoid of secretion. Occasional glands appear to have developed weak secretory activity. Spiral artery maturation is absent. Haematoxylin and Eosin × 117.

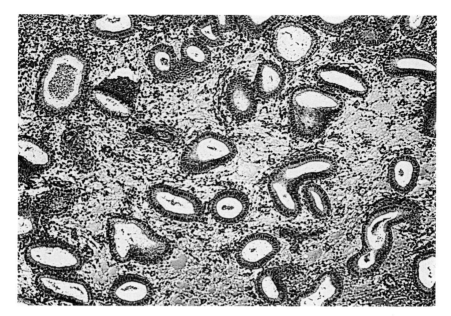

Figure 4.6 Luteal phase insufficiency, 26th day of a 28 day cycle. The endometrial glands are narrow with parallel sides similar to those seen in the proliferative phase (Figure 2.9). There is evidence of secretion in occasional glands but the general morphology contrasts sharply with that seen in Figure 3.18, which was taken only 24 hours later in a normal cycle. Haematoxylin and Eosin × 93.

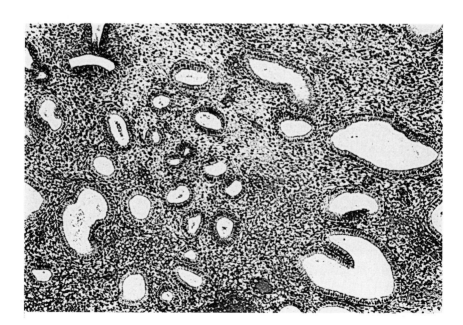

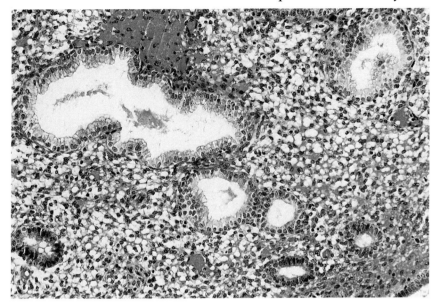

Figure 4.8   Luteal phase insufficiency, irregular ripening. This is a sample from a woman of 35 years who complained of almost continuous irregular spotting. There is a marked discrepancy between the maturation of the weakly secretory gland above and the small inactive glands below. Haematoxylin and Eosin × 186.

and undistended, even 8 or 9 days after ovulation, and secretion in the glandular lumina is scanty (Figure 4.5). Spiral arteries appear few in number and their growth is poorly developed.

When preceding oestrogen levels have been normal, luteal insufficiency may be characterized by a generally poor, delayed glandular secretory transformation (Figure 4.6) with narrow, straight or only mildly convoluted glands undistended by, or containing only a little, secretion, or by glands showing variation in maturation. In the latter case, sometimes also termed irregular ripening, glands which exhibit weak secretion, show normal secretion for the stage of the cycle, are inactive or show proliferative activity may co-exist (Figures 4.7 and 4.8). In a hysterectomy specimen it is possible, in some cases, to see that the most

Figure 4.7   Luteal phase insufficiency, irregular ripening, day 22 to 23 of a 28 day cycle. There is a marked difference between the small, unresponsive glands in the centre of the field and the surrounding glands which show moderate secretory activity. Haematoxylin and Eosin × 93.

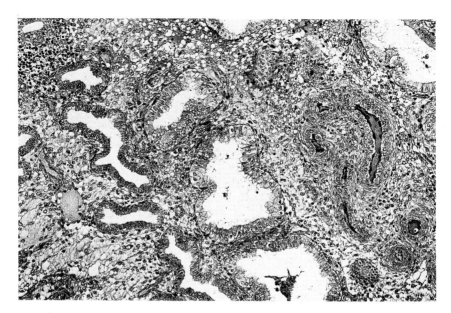

Figure 4.9 Luteal phase insufficiency, irregular ripening. The glands exhibiting the most adequate secretory transformation lie adjacent to the spiral artery whilst the gland furthest away (to the left) shows only very weak secretory activity. Note the well-developed spiral artery. Haematoxylin and Eosin × 149.

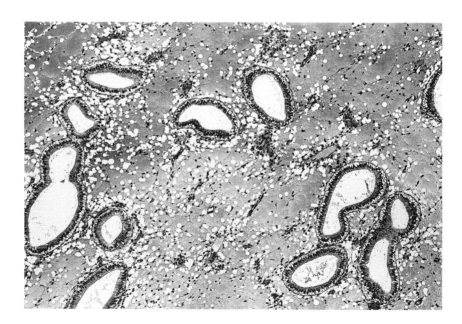

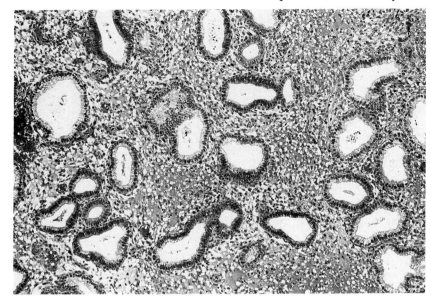

Figure 4.11   Luteal phase insufficiency, 22nd day of a 28 day cycle. Glandular secretion is rather weak, spiral artery development is negligible and the stroma is immature. Haematoxylin and Eosin × 117.

mature glands lie in proximity to the spiral arteries whilst the least well-developed glands lie at the greatest distance from these vessels (Figures 4.4–4.9). This phenomenon is rarely apparent in a biopsy. The stroma may be relatively more oedematous than in the normal cycle and the stromal cells, which depend upon progesterone for their maturation to predecidual cells, may be immature (Figure 4.10). Spiral arteries, which also depend upon progesterone for their differentiation, appear few in number and poorly differentiated (Figure 4.11).

Luteal phase insufficiency with oestrogen predominance is common. The endometrium is thick and well-grown and biopsies therefore ample. The stroma remains cellular and rich in fibroblasts, though lacking in collagen even many days after ovulation. The glands are numerous,

---

Figure 4.10   Luteal phase insufficiency, delayed secretory transformation, 21st day of a 27 to 28 day cycle. The glands are consistent in appearance with the 3rd post-ovulatory day and appear uniformly secretory. The stroma is immature and excessively oedematous for the 21st day of the cycle. Haematoxylin and Eosin × 93.

somewhat dilated and regular or slightly convoluted. Mitoses may persist in the glandular epithelium, which can be stratified, and glycogen secretion co-exists as basal and apical vacuoles. Spiral arteries are thick-walled and well-differentiated (Figures 4.12 and 4.13). The picture is that of delayed endometrial glandular maturation with a discrepancy between the stromal and glandular maturation.

In those endometria in which there is a discrepancy between the maturation of the glands and stroma, glandular secretion may be uniformly weak, irregular or just delayed whilst stromal maturation, in terms of stromal decidualization and spiral artery differentiation, is in advance of the glandular maturation (Figure 4.12). The discrepancy may vary from 2 to 7 or more days and examination of the spiral arteries is the single most useful diagnostic clue in these cases. The reason for the usefulness of the spiral artery maturation in identifying the actual date of the cycle lies in the fact that spiral artery differentiation is exquisitely sensitive to progesterone and occurs in response to only a minute quantity of progesterone in the presence of only moderate or even slight oestrogenic stimulation (de Brux, 1981b).

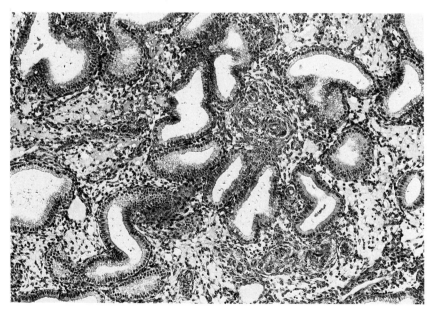

Figure 4.12   Luteal phase insufficiency, 23rd to 24th day of a 28 day cycle. Spiral arteries are well muscularized and surrounded by a cuff of predecidual cells which is consistent with the date of the cycle. In contrast the glands are narrow and weakly secretory, approximately equivalent in activity to the 5th post-ovulatory day. Haematoxylin and Eosin × 117.

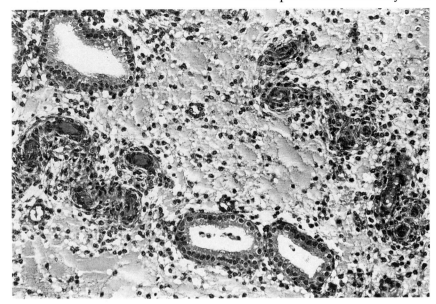

Figure 4.13   Luteal phase insufficiency, 23rd day of a 28 to 29 day cycle. The spiral artery maturation corresponds to the day of the cycle but the glands are very narrow and only very weakly secretory. Haematoxylin and Eosin × 186.

4.3.3   *Premature failure of the corpus luteum*

Premature failure of the corpus luteum leads to a short luteal phase, and is sometimes encountered in patients complaining of premenstrual bleeding or spotting, or infertility. It is recognized in a biopsy by the finding of focal interstitial stromal haemorrhage and crumbling, indicative of tissue breakdown, in an endometrium which is either not fully mature or exhibits the features described above as characterizing luteal phase insufficiency. In the absence of stromal crumbling, stromal mitoses prior to the 12th post-ovulatory day, which mark a return of oestrogen dominance, may indicate failure of the corpus luteum.

4.3.4   *Delayed, prolonged or irregular shedding*

In some patients, in whom there has been a premature decline in progesterone secretion, shedding of the endometrium may not only commence early but also take longer than normal and may be associated with persistence of a functional corpus luteum. Such cases are recognized by the presence, in uterine curettings, of secretory endometrium several

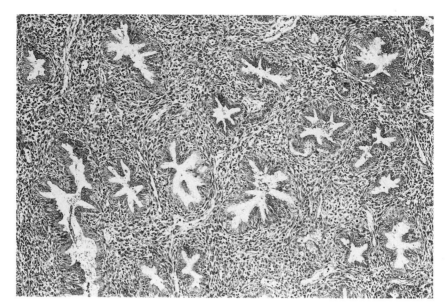

Figure 4.14 Delayed endometrial shedding. The stellate glands set in a fibrous stroma infiltrated by lymphocytes are typical of this state. This patient had been bleeding for two weeks at the time of the biopsy. Haematoxylin and Eosin × 93.

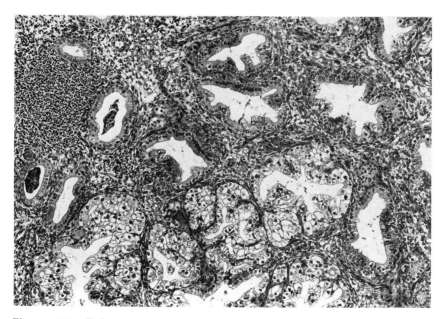

Figure 4.15 Delayed endometrial shedding. Glands exhibiting Arias-Stella change (lower part of the field) are visible in this curettage sample from a woman who had had a spontaneous abortion two weeks earlier. Haematoxylin and Eosin × 117.

days after the onset of bleeding. The secretory endometrium in these cases may retain features of the luteal phase insufficiency, but if the endometrium had previously been of normal apperance this will also be apparent. In the latter case the sample most commonly consists of fragments of endometrium that have undergone regression and shrinkage rather than fragmentation and disintegration (Dallenbach-Hellweg and Bornebusch, 1970). These tend to have a rather fibrous stroma, sometimes infiltrated by a scattering of chronic inflammatory cells, and the glands have a stellate outline in transverse section (Figure 4.14). A similar phenomenon is also encountered in patients having a spontaneous abortion and it is one of the common appearances observed in endometrium removed at curettage following a miscarriage (Figure 4.15) (Chapter 13).

In certain women, in whom there is delayed or prolonged shedding, endometrial regrowth may occur before shedding is complete and in these circumstances, curettage or biopsy material may contain a mixture of secretory endometrium, showing the features of delayed shedding, menstrual type fragments and proliferative endometrium (Figure 4.16).

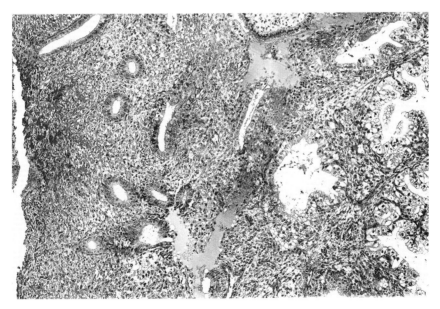

Figure 4.16   Delayed shedding. Both hypersecretory endometrium (to the right) and proliferative endometrium (to the left) are present in this curettage sample from a woman who had been bleeding for 12 days. It is likely that she had had a spontaneous abortion. Haematoxylin and Eosin × 93.

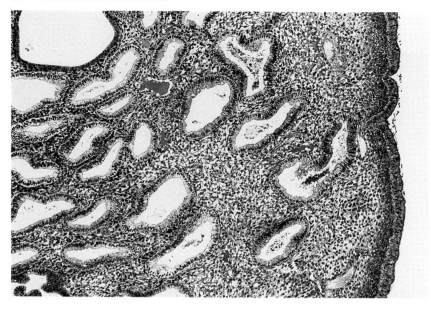

Figure 4.17 This is a biopsy from an infertile woman in whom luteal phase insufficiency had been reported in previous cycles. In view of the failure to develop an adequate secretory endometrium Norethisterone had been given in this cycle, 8 days before the biopsy. Notice the very poor response to this therapy. Haematoxylin and Eosin × 93.

4.3.5   Progesterone receptor defect

Occasionally the endometrial appearance suggests luteal phase insufficiency yet hormonal secretion patterns are normal. It can be demonstrated that such endometria contain fewer high affinity progesterone binding sites in the cytosol fraction of the endometrium than normal (Figure 4.17) (Cooke *et al.*, 1972; Keller *et al.*, 1979; Laatikainen *et al.*, 1983).

References

Cooke, I.D., Morgan, C.A. and Parry, I.E. (1972) Correlation of endometrial biopsy and plasma progesterone levels in infertile women. *J. Obstet. Gynaecol. Br. Cwlth*, **79**, 647–50.

Dallenbach-Hellweg, G. (1987) Functional disturbances of the endometrium. In *Haines and Taylor: Obstetrical and Gynaecological Pathology* (ed. H. Fox), Churchill-Livingstone, Edinburgh, pp. 320–39.

Dallenbach-Hellweg, G. and Bornebusch, C.G. (1970) Histologische Untersuchungen über die Reaction des Endometrium bei der verzögerten Abstossung. *Arch. Gynäkol.*, **208**, 234–46.

de Brux, J. (1981a) Evaluation of ovarian disturbances by endometrial biopsy. In *The Endometrium. Hormonal Impacts* (eds J. de Brux, R. Mortel and J.P. Gautray), Plenum Press, New York and London, pp. 107–21.

de Brux, J. (1981b) Analysis of isolated and combined sections of ovarian steroids on the endometrium. In *The Endometrium. Hormonal Impacts* (eds J. de Brux, R. Mortel and J.P. Gautray), Plenum Press, New York and London, pp. 31–42.

Keller, D.W., Wiest, W.G., Askin, F.B., Johnson, L.W. and Strickler, R.C. (1979) Pseudocorpus luteum insufficiency: a local defect of progesterone action on endometrial tissue. *J. Clin. Endocrinol. Metabol.*, **48**, 127–32.

Laatikainen, T., Andersson, B., Kärkkäinen, J. and Wahlström, T. (1983) Progestin receptor levels in endometria with delayed or incomplete secretory changes. *Obstet. Gynecol.*, **62**, 592–8.

5 The effect of therapeutic and contraceptive hormones on the endometrium

Exogenous sex steroid hormones may be administered to a woman for contraceptive or therapeutic purposes or as replacements for diminished or absent endogenous hormones. Such hormones markedly influence endometrial histology and their use, particularly for contraceptive purposes, is now so widespread that a pathologist required to interpret endometrial biopsies must insist upon receiving a history which includes details of recent, and not simply current, exposure of the patient to exogenous steroids. In the absence of such a history the pathologist is, to a significant extent, working in the dark.

In patients receiving exogenous hormones for either replacement or therapeutic purposes the endometrium is commonly biopsied in order to monitor the morphological changes induced in the endometrium or, in some instances, the response of the disease which is being treated. By contrast, endometrial biopsies in women using steroids for contraceptive purposes are almost invariably undertaken for purposes unrelated to their hormone usage and it is particularly under these circumstances that the pathologist may, in the absence of a reliable contraceptive history, be led astray.

5.1 The effects of hormonal therapy

5.1.1 Oestrogens

Oestrogens are given for the relief of menopausal symptoms, as post-menopausal hormone replacement therapy, or as a factor in the management of hypogonadal conditions, e.g. gonadal dysgenesis.

Oestrogens normally affect synchronous growth of the endometrial glands, stroma and vasculature, induce endometrial progesterone receptors and, in the normal cycle, cause the stromal oedema which characterizes the mid-secretory phase. The endometrial morphological response to exogenous hormones, however, depends not only upon the duration of administration of oestrogen, the potency of the hormonal preparation and the total dosage but also upon the endogenous hormonal status of the patient.

If oestrogens are given to a woman who is in the proliferative phase of the cycle endometrial growth is prolonged, and the endometrium may exhibit features of a prolonged proliferative phase (Chapter 4); ovulation is suppressed or delayed and the secretory phase is shortened or absent (Dallenbach-Hellweg, 1981). Oestrogen administration during the secretory phase results in marked stromal oedema, incomplete secretory transformation of the glands and retarded stromal maturation (Egger and Kinderman, 1980), a picture which resembles that of spontaneous luteal phase insufficiency.

More commonly, of course, oestrogens are given to women with a paucity of endogenous hormone, an absence of cyclical changes and an atrophic endometrium. Under these circumstances small doses of oestrogen induce only a weakly proliferative pattern with a few visible mitoses, a poorly defined functionalis and relatively little thickening of the endometrium; there may be focal multilayering of the glandular epithelium (Figure 5.1). If dosage at this level is given for a prolonged

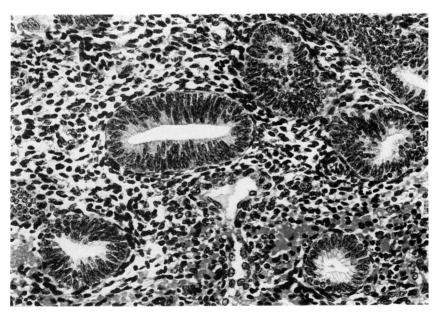

Figure 5.1 Weakly proliferative endometrium in a woman presenting with postmenopausal bleeding six years after the menopause. She had been treated intermittently with small doses of unopposed oestrogen. Epithelial stratification is present but the stroma remains compact. Haematoxylin and Eosin × 370.

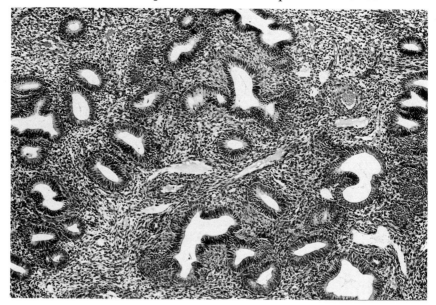

Figure 5.2   Disordered proliferation. A minor degree of glandular architectural irregularity is present in the endometrium of a woman treated with unopposed oestrogen for many years after the menopause. Haematoxylin and Eosin × 93.

period the glands may eventually show a minor degree of dilatation and architectural atypia (Figures 5.2 and 5.3), the appearances being those of a 'disordered proliferative endometrium' (Chapters 4 and 9) (Hendrickson and Kempson, 1980). In patients given higher physiological doses of oestrogen, either continuously or cyclically, a significant proportion will develop either a simple, complex or atypical endometrial hyperplasia, if a progestagen is not also given (Whitehead *et al.*, 1977; Campenhout *et al.*, 1980; Fox and Buckley, 1982; Schiff *et al.*, 1982) (Chapter 9). A much smaller proportion of women on long-term oestrogen dosage will eventually develop an endometrial carcinoma, albeit one which is usually of the well-differentiated endometrioid type. If a progestagen is administered with the oestrogen, either in combination or sequentially, both hyperplasia and adenocarcinoma will be prevented and any hyperplastic process which has developed during unopposed oestrogenic stimulation will often be reversed.

5.1.2   *Tamoxifen*

Tamoxifen is a triphenylethylene compound which, as a consequence of competing for and blocking oestrogen binding sites, has anti-oestrogenic

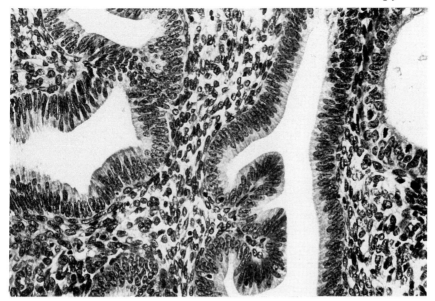

Figure 5.3   Disordered proliferation. Glandular epithelium is similar to that seen in the weakly proliferative endometrium (Figure 5.1) and in the basalis of the reproductive years (Figure 3.6). There is no cytological atypia and epithelial stratification is minimal. A mitosis is present in the gland to the right. Haematoxylin and Eosin × 370.

properties. It is convenient to consider its effects here, however, because in a small proportion of women it appears, somewhat paradoxically, to induce an oestrogen-like effect. This has been described both experimentally, when the drug has been used at a level exceeding the recommended dose by over 100 times, and clinically at therapeutic levels (Legault-Poisson *et al.*, 1979).

The effects of Tamoxifen on the endometrium may amount to no more than epithelial multilayering but it can induce proliferative activity or hyperplasia in women receiving treatment for breast carcinoma (Figure 5.4). We have also seen a case of endometrial carcinoma where there was no other clear aetiological factor and the suspicion remains that it may have been Tamoxifen-driven. The patient was a postmenopausal woman being treated for breast carcinoma by Tamoxifen; she had no other apparent oestrogenic source. We have also observed a dramatic response to norethisterone following Tamoxifen therapy, indicating that progesterone receptors had been induced.

Oestrogenic effects may, therefore, be observed in endometrial biopsies from patients receiving this form of therapy.

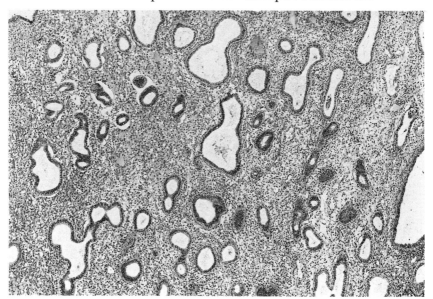

Figure 5.4   Mild simple hyperplasia in an endometrium from a patient who had received Tamoxifen for the treatment of breast carcinoma until 14 days before the biopsy. Haematoxylin and Eosin × 60.

More commonly, Tamoxifen is used to suppress ovulation temporarily in the treatment of infertility with the intention of causing 'rebound' ovulation when the drug is withdrawn. The endometrium from such patients may exhibit a wide variety of appearances, both prior to treatment and following therapy.

5.1.3   Progestagens

Progestagens are used in the management of dysfunctional uterine bleeding, endometriosis, endometrial hyperplasia and some cases of endometrial adenocarcinoma. They act only on an endometrium in which progesterone receptors have been induced by prior exposure to oestrogen, exert an anti-oestrogenic effect with inhibition of endometrial growth and also induce differentiation or maturation of the glands and stroma.

When progestagens are given in therapeutic doses to a patient, the appearances of her endometrium will depend upon the extent to which the endometrium has been primed by oestrogen and upon the biochemical characteristics of the particular hormone. If progestagens are given early in the proliferative phase little stromal decidualization occurs

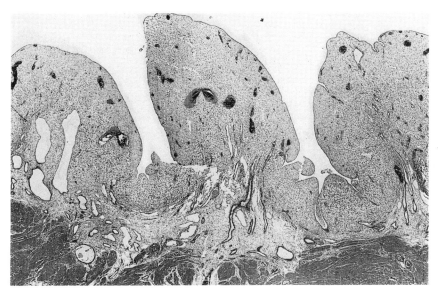

Figure 5.5 Progestagen therapy. The polypoidal appearance which the endometrium assumes following treatment by Norethisterone. Note the marked pseudodecidualization of the superficial part of the stroma, the paucity of glands and the congested thin-walled blood vessels. Haematoxylin and Eosin × 18.5.

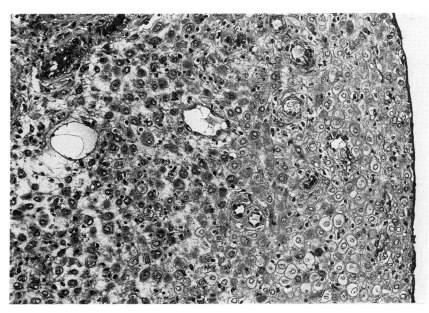

Figure 5.6 Progestagen therapy. The florid pseudodecidualization of the endometrial stroma which follows treatment with Norethisterone. Stromal cells are enlarged and have well-demarcated cell borders. Haematoxylin and Eosin × 186.

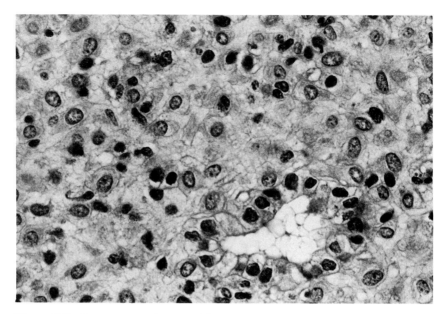

Figure 5.7 Progestagen therapy. The stroma is pseudodecidualized and the gland to the right is narrow and lined by inactive, cuboidal clear cells. K-cells are scattered throughout the stroma. Haematoxylin and Eosin × 750.

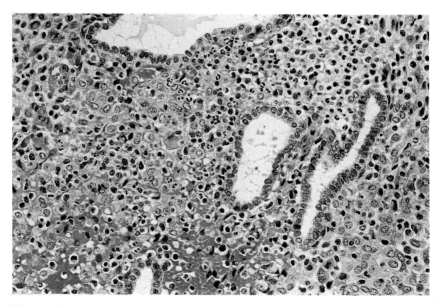

Figure 5.8 Progestagen withdrawal bleeding. The stroma in the centre of the field is undergoing necrosis and there is focal haemorrhage. An infiltrate of polymorphonuclear leucocytes contrasts with the K-cells seen in Figure 5.7. Note the inactivity of the glands. Haematoxylin and Eosin × 297.

and there may be only a minor degree of abortive secretory activity in glands that remain narrow and tubular. Spiral artery differentiation is not seen. The administration of a progestagen to a patient late in the proliferative phase will induce marked pseudodecidualization of the functionalis (Figures 5.5 and 5.6) and transitory glandular secretory activity, reflecting the widespread prior induction of progesterone receptors. The glands rapidly exhaust their secretory activity and become small and inactive though occasional glands may retain a secretory, or even hypersecretory, appearance. K-cells (granulated lymphocytes) are scattered throughout the decidualized stroma and these may form small aggregates (Figure 5.7). It is important to distinguish these from polymorphonuclear leucocytes which they may, at first glance, resemble (Figure 5.8). This pattern can be confused with that of early pregnancy in which the glands are, at least focally, hypersecretory and there is good growth of the spiral arteries (Figures 13.1 and 13.2).

Prolonged progestagen therapy results in an atrophic endometrium with sparse glands set in a shallow, compact stroma; the glands are

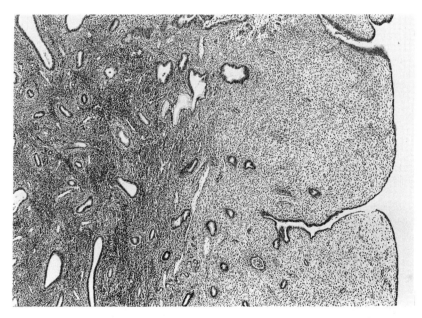

Figure 5.9 Prolonged progestagen therapy, moderate atrophy. Endometrial depth is much reduced, the marked polypoidal appearance associated with the recent commencement of progestagen is not seen. There is a shallow functionalis with pseudodecidualized stroma almost devoid of glands and most glands are inactive. Spiral arteries are not differentiated. Haematoxylin and Eosin × 47.

76   The effect of therapeutic and contraceptive hormones

inactive, though their epithelium may remain columnar rather than cuboidal (Figure 5.9). It is usual for the K-cell infiltrate to persist whilst thin-walled vascular channels of indeterminate type are a conspicuous feature (Figure 5.10), these possibly being the source of the intermittent breakthrough bleeding experienced by these patients. Spiral artery growth is absent. Endometrial atrophy of this type, which is due to the antioestrogenic effect of the progestagens, will persist as long as the progestagen therapy is continued but usually recovers rapidly after withdrawal of the exogenous hormone. Permanent atrophy with stromal hyalinization has been described (Dallenbach-Hellweg, 1980) but is, in practice, very rarely encountered.

The appearances described above are seen most markedly in women receiving 19-nortestosterone-derived progestagens. In women given the weakly progestagenic synthetic anti-gonadotrophic androgen Danol (Danazol), used particularly in the treatment of endometriosis, a moderately atrophic endometrium lacking stromal decidualization and glandular secretory activity develops rapidly *ab initio* (Figure 5.11).

In women treated with progestagens for dysfunctional uterine bleeding

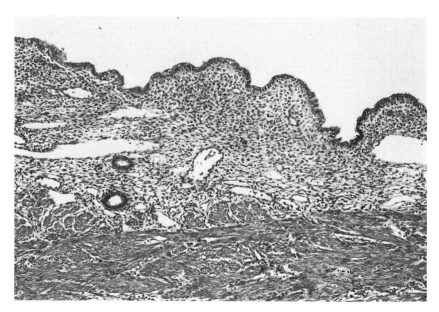

Figure 5.10   Prolonged progestagen therapy with profound atrophy. The uterus is lined only by a shallow, inactive endometrium containing narrow tubular glands and thin-walled vascular channels. Vascular and stromal differentiation are absent. There is no functionalis. Haematoxylin and Eosin × 93.

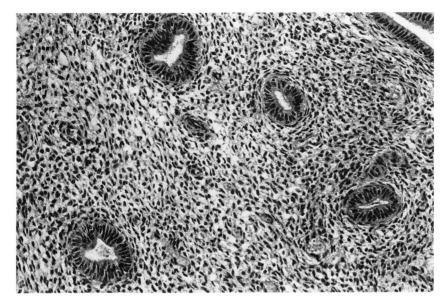

Figure 5.11 Danazol therapy. The endometrial glands are narrow, tubular and inactive and the stroma is immature and spindle-celled. The appearances are similar to those seen following prolonged treatment with Norethisterone. Haematoxylin and Eosin × 232.

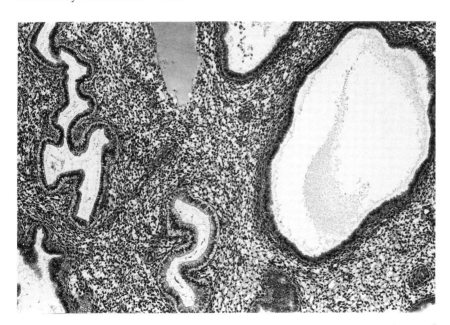

Figure 5.12 Progestagen therapy. Patchy, weak secretory activity superimposed on a simple hyperplasia. The patient had been treated with Norethisterone. Haematoxylin and Eosin × 93.

the typical changes described above are commonly seen. However, in some cases of dysfunctional uterine bleeding there is an underlying endometrial hyperplasia, upon which secretory changes may be superimposed (Figures 5.12 and 5.13), this appearance sometimes being called 'secretory hyperplasia', an unnecessary and potentially misleading term. With continued therapy simple hyperplasia may regress completely but atypical hyperplasia may regress only partly, leaving islands of architecturally atypical glands set in an endometrium which is otherwise relatively normal in appearance, pseudo-decidualized or possibly atrophic (Figure 5.14).

Hormonally responsive endometrial adenocarcinomas, which are usually well-differentiated (Grade 1) tumours, may also show secretory changes within 10 to 14 days of commencing progestagen therapy (Figure 10.11) whilst the stromal cells of the neoplasm can show pseudodecidualization (Ferenczy, 1980). Tumour growth may be suppressed and focal areas of regression or degeneration may be apparent (Anderson, 1972; Rosier and Underwood, 1974; Dallenbach-Hellweg, 1980; Ferenczy, 1980).

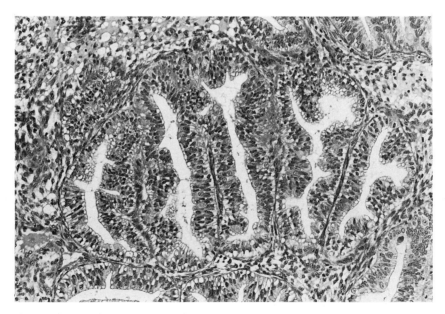

Figure 5.13 Progestagen therapy. Secretory transformation superimposed on an endometrium with the features of complex hyperplasia. Uniform subnuclear vacuoles are present in the glandular epithelial cells. Haematoxylin and Eosin × 186.

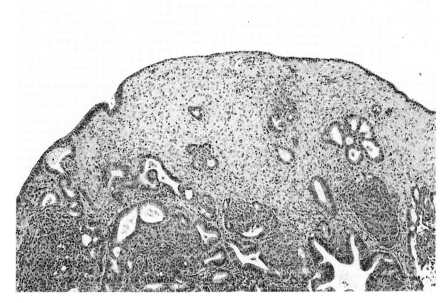

Figure 5.14 Progestagen therapy, persistent atypical hyperplasia. The stroma is pseudodecidualized and the glands in the superficial part of the tissue are narrow and tubular, those in the deeper part remain architecturally and cytologically atypical and many contain foci of squamous metaplasia. Haematoxylin and Eosin × 93.

5.2 The effects of contraceptive hormones

Steroid contraceptives fall into two main groups, those in which an oestrogen and progestagen are given in combination and those containing only a progestagen.

Most women follow a regimen in which between 20 and 50 μg of oestrogen, usually ethinyloestradiol, combined with a progestagen is taken for 21 days out of every 28. The proportion of hormone in the preparation may be identical throughout the 21 days or there may be a phased formulation in which the hormone content of the pill is increased in the middle of the cycle. It is usual to commence therapy on the first day of the cycle as it has been shown that by postponing the commencement to the 5th day, as was previously recommended, ovulation may not be inhibited in the first cycle. On the 7 hormone-free days either a placebo is taken or there are 7 pill-free days.

Some women, particularly those over the age of 35 years, heavy smokers and those in whom oestrogens induce severe side-effects, may use a progestagen-only contraceptive. The progestagen, which is taken every day, may be administered in several ways, the effects upon the endometrium being independent of the mode of administration.

5.2.1   Combined steroid contraceptives

In the first few months in which a combined steroid contraceptive is used, the pattern of endometrial changes may be cyclical but after prolonged usage the regenerative capacity of the endometrium may be diminished, because of progestagen predominance, and an atrophic picture ensues (Figure 5.15). The morphological effects of combined steroid contraceptives, whilst being generally similar whatever the precise hormone combination and dosage, show sufficient variation for the relative importance of the oestrogen and progestagen in the combination to be recognized and for this to be associated in some patients with particular problems.

Following hormonal withdrawal bleeding at the end of each cycle of hormone usage (Figure 5.16), the endometrium regenerates and there is a proliferative phase which is curtailed by the inhibitory effect of the progestagen upon the oestrogen stimulated growth, the endometrium

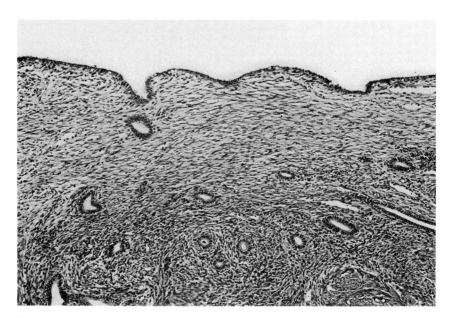

Figure 5.15   Long-term combined steroid contraceptive, biphasic pattern. The endometrium is moderately atrophic and resembles that seen in progestagen users (Figure 5.9). The patient had used a combination of 30 μg of ethinyloestradiol with 150 μg of levonorgestrel. Haematoxylin and Eosin × 117.

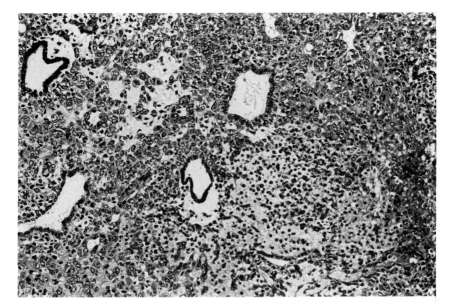

Figure 5.16 Combined steroid contraceptive, biphasic pattern. Hormone withdrawal bleeding on the second day of the cycle. The glands are small and inactive, there is no evidence of secretory change and the stroma is crumbling and haemorrhagic. Contrast with the appearance of menstrual endometrium (Figure 3.8). Haematoxylin and Eosin × 186.

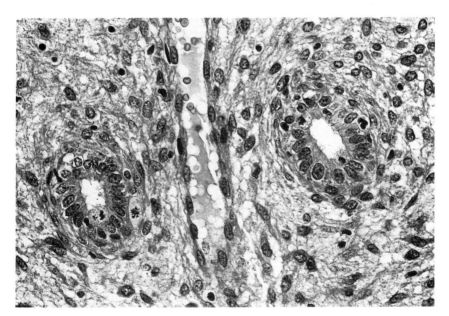

Figure 5.17 Combined steroid contraceptive, biphasic pattern, 8th day of the cycle, the proliferative phase. Mitoses are present in both the glandular epithelium and in the stroma. Haematoxylin and Eosin × 465.

therefore remaining shallow. The glands, which are narrow, sometimes extremely so, lack the tortuosity of the normal proliferative phase and may appear sparse. They are lined by a single layer of cubo-columnar cells in which a small number of mitoses are seen (Figure 5.17). The stromal cells, in which only occasional mitoses appear, remain spindled and have the so-called 'naked-nucleus' appearance.

Between the 8th and 10th day of the cycle, the progestagen effect becomes apparent and subnuclear vacuoles appear in the glandular epithelial cells (Figure 5.18) but, because of the brief, inadequate oestrogenic priming, progestagen receptors are few in number and the secretory changes are weak and poorly developed. By day 10 the subnuclear secretory vacuoles move into the supranuclear cytoplasm and there is a short, premature secretory phase lasting until day 14 or 15. The glands remain narrow, or only minimally dilated, and straight or only gently convoluted. The cytoplasm of the glandular epithelium, which is columnar, appears faintly eosinophilic. The apices of the cells remain, for the most part, intact and there is only a trace of secretion within the lumina (Figure 5.19). There is, in some patients, a little stromal oedema. In the latter half of the cycle there is regression of secretory change and

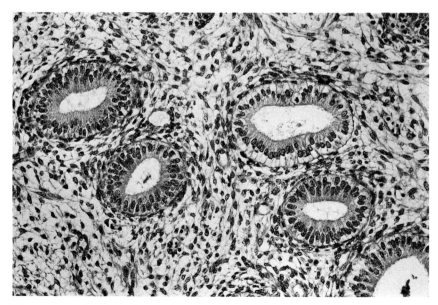

Figure 5.18   Combined steroid contraceptive, 8th day of the cycle in a phased contraceptive user. Subnuclear vacuoles are present in all the glands and there is a resemblance to the early secretory phase of the physiological cycle. Gland size, however, remains small. Haematoxylin and Eosin × 232.

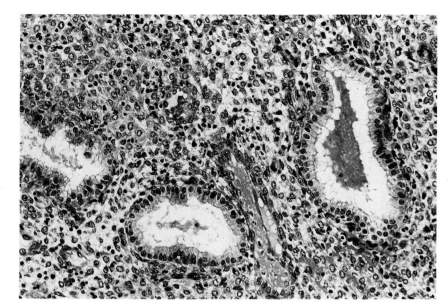

Figure 5.19 Combined steroid contraceptive, biphasic pattern. A weak secretory transformation with poor vascular differentiation. A sprinkling of K-cells is present. Haematoxylin and Eosin × 232.

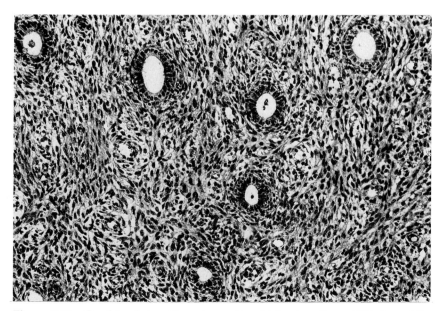

Figure 5.20 Combined steroid contraceptive, biphasic pattern, 24th day of the cycle. The glands are extremely narrow and inactive and the stroma densely cellular with a pseudodecidualized appearance. Haematoxylin and Eosin × 186.

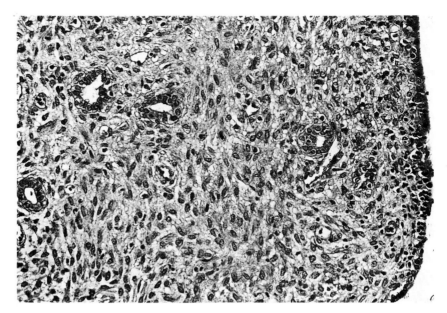

Figure 5.21 Combined steroid contraceptive, biphasic pattern, 50 mg ethinyloestradiol, 250 mg levonorgesterel, 26th day of the cycle. The glands are extremely narrow and inactive, the stroma is markedly pseudodecidualized, forming a compacta, and there is a K-cell infiltrate. Haematoxylin and Eosin × 232.

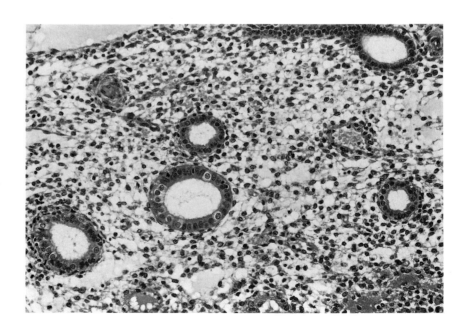

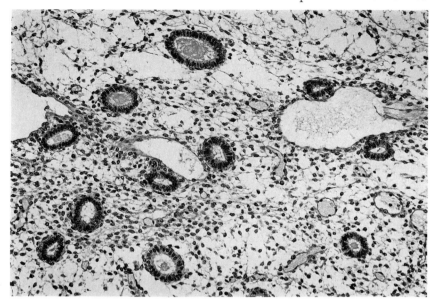

Figure 5.23 Combined steroid contraceptive, biphasic pattern, 35 mg ethinyloestradiol, 1 mg Norethisterone. The glands are small and inactive, the stroma is immature and there is no spiral artery differentiation; thin-walled vascular channels are present. The appearances are similar to those seen in Figure 5.22. Haematoxylin and Eosin × 186.

the endometrium becomes inactive (Figure 5.20). The degree of spiral artery differentiation and growth, the quality of stromal pseudo-decidualization and the extent of the glandular secretory transformation vary according to the relative potency of the oestrogen and progestagen in the combination (Buckley, 1987) and the duration of use (Figures 5.21 to 5.24).

The alternating nodules of stromal hyperplasia and oedema described by Dallenbach-Hellweg (1981) and the bizarre stromal pseudo-sarcomatous changes reported by Dockerty et al. (1959) are not, in our experience, encountered in users of modern, low dose, steroid contraceptives.

Figure 5.22 Combined steroid contraceptive, biphasic pattern, 30 mg ethinyloestradiol, 250 mg levonorgesterel, three weeks since hormone withdrawal bleeding. In comparison with Figure 5.21, the glands are less atrophic and the stroma is immature; there is no decidualization. Haematoxylin and Eosin × 232.

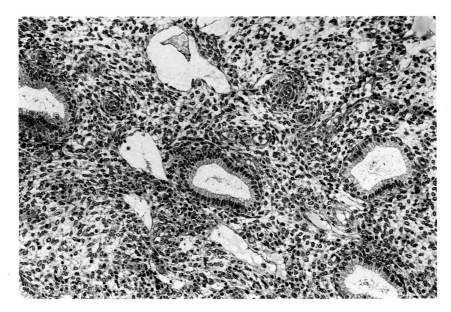

Figure 5.24 Combined steroid contraceptive, biphasic pattern, 30 mg ethinyloestradiol, 150 mg levonorgesterel, three weeks since hormone withdrawal bleeding. In contrast to the three preceding illustrations, the glands are moderately well-grown, exhibit secretory activity and spiral artery differentiation has occurred. A K-cell infiltrate is present. Haematoxylin and Eosin × 186.

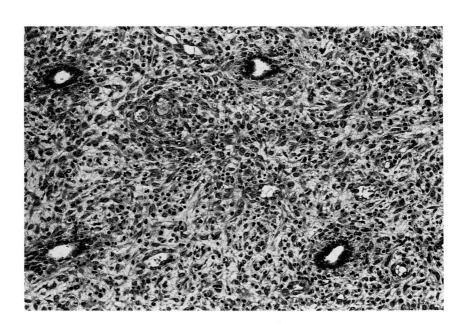

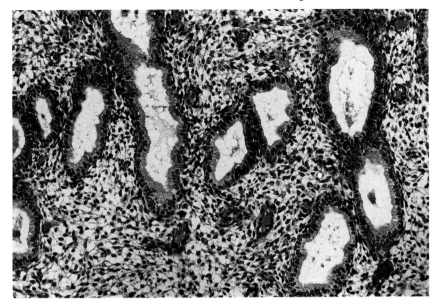

Figure 5.26 Phased steroid contraceptive. This biopsy was from a patient receiving a hormone combination identical to that given to the woman whose biopsy appears in Figure 5.25. In striking contrast glandular growth and secretion are much better developed, there is a minor degree of spiral artery differentiation and K-cell infiltration is absent. Haematoxylin and Eosin × 186.

The appearances observed after the 15th day of the cycle are more variable in users of the phased contraceptives. In some patients a picture indistinguishable from that seen in conventional combined steroid contraceptive users is observed (Figure 5.25) whilst in others there is less glandular regression, a persistence of weak secretory activity to the time of withdrawal and, in those preparations with increased midcycle oestrogen and hence more adequate progestagen receptor induction, better growth and muscularization of the spiral arteries (Figure 5.26).

We do not currently encounter women using sequential steroid contraceptives in which a period of oestrogen therapy is followed by a short phase of a progestagen-oestrogen combination.

Figure 5.25   Phased steroid contraceptive. The glands are small, narrow, tubular and devoid of secretion. The stroma is pseudodecidualized and infiltrated by K-cells. The degree of glandular regression is similar to that seen in Figure 5.21. Haematoxylin and Eosin × 186.

88　The effect of therapeutic and contraceptive hormones

In contrast to patients receiving oestrogen therapy, women using combined steroid contraceptives are protected against the risk of developing endometrial carcinoma, having only half the risk compared with 'never-users' (Huggins and Giuntoli, 1979; Kaufman *et al.*, 1980; Weiss and Sayvetz, 1980; Hulka *et al.*, 1982; WHO, 1982). This beneficial effect persists after the menopause providing the woman is not given unopposed oestrogen replacement therapy. Maximum protection is afforded to those who are nulliparous and have used the pill for more than one year.

5.2.1　Progestagen-only contraceptives

A very variable endometrial picture is encountered in women using a progestagen-only contraceptive. The dose is small and its contraceptive effect depends not upon suppression of ovulation but upon alterations in tubal transport and in the quality of the cervical mucus. Ovulation is suppressed in only about 50% of cycles and as a consequence the

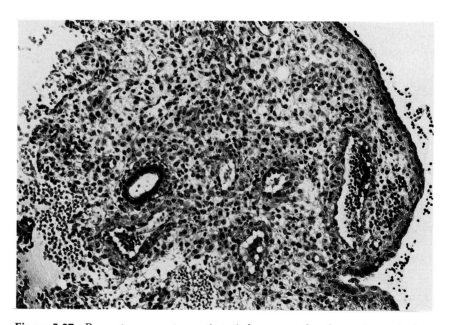

Figure 5.27　Progestagen contraceptive. A fragment of endometrium which is typical of that obtained from a woman using a depot progestagen for contraceptive purposes. A single inactive gland and several abnormal, dilated vascular channels are present. Haematoxylin and Eosin × 186.

underlying endogenous hormone pattern may vary from cycle to cycle and from patient to patient. In addition it is usual to give the same dose of progestagen every day, or administer it systemically by depot injection, rather than in a cyclical pattern, and amenorrhoea or breakthrough bleeding with intermittent healing therefore occurs.

The most commonly encountered pattern is one in which glands of rather variable size and secretory activity are set in a spindle-celled stroma containing thin-walled vascular channels and showing little or no evidence of decidualization (Figures 5.27 and 5.28). The appearances are reminiscent of those sometimes encountered in luteal phase insufficiency. If bleeding has occurred recently mitoses may be seen in both glandular epithelium and stromal cells and if ovulation has occurred there may be sufficient proliferative activity both to increase the general thickness of the endometrium and to permit spiral artery growth and muscularization. The appearances do not resemble those seen in patients receiving high doses of progestagen for therapeutic purposes (see above).

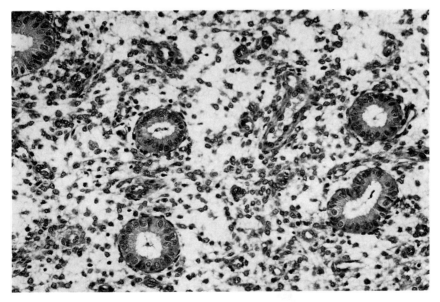

Figure 5.28   Progestagen contraceptive, daily dose of 0.35 mg of Norethisterone. The appearance of the endometrium in progestagen-only contraceptive users is very variable, in this case it resembles that seen in Figures 5.22 and 5.23 in which combinations with relatively high doses of progestagen have been taken. Spiral artery differentiation has not occurred, the glands are small and inactive and the stroma is immature. Haematoxylin and Eosin × 232.

5.3   Hormone replacement therapy

It is considered unwise to use oestrogens alone for replacement therapy
when the uterus is *in situ* because of the risk that endometrial carcinoma
may develop. None the less, from time to time we encounter patients in
whom this has occurred (Figures 5.2 and 5.3). More commonly, oestrogen
is given for between 10 and 15 days, on average, and then a progestagen
is added to the regime for the next 5 to 10 days. This eliminates the risk
of inducing endometrial carcinoma (Whitehead *et al.*, 1982). Other less
commonly used combinations include the combining of an oestrogen
with testosterone. We have not, however, had the opportunity of
examining the endometria of women using the latter regimen.

Following the administration of oestrogen, the endometrium
proliferates and grows normally for the first part of the treatment cycle
and after introduction of the progestagen there is a brief, poorly
developed, delayed secretory phase which may not appear until shortly
before hormonal withdrawal bleeding. There is little or no stromal

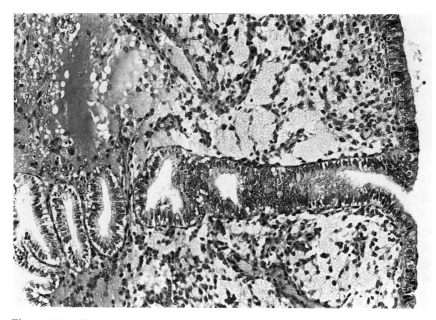

Figure 5.29   Hormone replacement therapy, sequential pattern. The sample was
taken on the 23rd day of an artificial 28 day cycle. The endometrium is well-grown
and there is subnuclear vacuolation of the glandular epithelium. Stromal oedema
is marked and spiral artery differentiation has not yet occurred. Haematoxylin
and Eosin × 186.

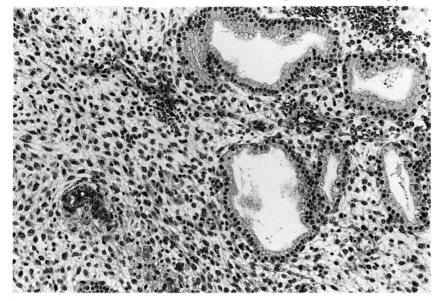

Figure 5.30 Hormone replacement therapy. Glands are well-grown, secretory activity is present, spiral artery differentiation has occurred and mild stromal pseudodecidualization has developed. Haematoxylin and Eosin × 186.

decidualization, though stromal oedema may be marked as a reflection of oestrogenic activity (Figure 5.29), and K-cells are sparse or absent. In a small proportion of women oestrogen is administered by means of a skin patch and progestagen is given either as an intramuscular depot injection or by mouth. In such cases, the endometrial appearances are variable, depending upon the dose and interval between administration of the two hormones and the biopsy. In many women endometrial morphology approximates to the normal, particularly in those in whom there has been premature ovarian failure (Figure 5.30).

Prolonged, balanced hormone replacement therapy has no adverse long-term consequences upon the endometrium of which we are aware and endometrial atrophy does not occur.

References

Anderson, D.G. (1972) The possible mechanisms of action of progestins on endometrial adenocarcinoma. *Am. J. Obstet. Gynecol.*, **113**, 195–211.

Buckley, C.H. (1987) Pathology of contraception and hormonal therapy. In *Haines and Taylor: Obstetrical and Gynaecological Pathology* (ed. H. Fox), Churchill Livingstone, Edinburgh, pp. 839–73.

Campenhout, J. van, Choquette, P. and Vauclair, R. (1980) Endometrial pattern in patients with primary hypoestrogenic amenorrhoea receiving estrogen replacement therapy. *Obstet. Gynecol.*, **56**, 349–55.

Dallenbach-Hellweg, G. (ed.) (1980) Morphological changes induced by exogenous gestagens in normal human endometrium. In *Functional Morphologic Changes in Female Sex Organs Induced by Exogenous Hormones*, Springer-Verlag, Berlin, Heidelberg, New York, pp. 95–100.

Dallenbach-Hellweg, G. (1981) *Histopathology of the Endometrium*, 3rd edn, Springer-Verlag, Berlin, Heidelberg, New York, pp. 126–256.

Dockerty, M.B., Smith, R.A. and Symmonds, R.E. (1959) Pseudomalignant endometrial changes induced by the administration of new synthetic progestins. *Proc. May Clinic.*, **34**, 321–8.

Egger, H. and Kinderman, G. (1980) Effects of high oestrogen doses on the endometrium. In *Functional Morphologic Changes in Female Sex Organs Induced by Exogenous Hormones* (ed. G. Dallenbach-Hellweg), Springer-Verlag, Berlin, Heidelberg, New York, pp. 51–3.

Ferenczy, A. (1980) Morphological effects of exogenous gestagens on abnormal human endometrium. In *Functional Morphologic Changes in Female Sex Organs Induced by Exogenous Hormones* (ed. G. Dallenbach-Hellweg), Springer-Verlag, Berlin, Heidelberg, New York, pp. 101–10.

Fox, H. and Buckley, C.H. (1982) The endometrial hyperplasias and their relationship to neoplasia. *Histopathology*, **6**, 493–510.

Hendrickson, M.R. and Kempson, R.L. (1980) *Surgical Pathology of the Uterine Corpus*, W.B. Saunders, Philadelphia, London, Toronto

Huggins, G.R. and Giuntoli, R.L. (1979) Oral contraceptives and neoplasia. *Fertil. Steril.*, **32**, 1–23.

Hulka, B.S., Chambless, L.E., Kaufman, D.G., Fowler, W.C. and Greenberg, B.G. (1982) Protection against endometrial carcinoma by combination-product oral contraceptives. *J. Am. Med. Ass.*, **247**, 475–7.

Kaufman, D.W., Shapiro, S., Slone, D. *et al.* (1980) Decreased risk of endometrial cancer among oral contraceptive users. *New Eng. J. Med.*, **303**, 1045–7.

Legault-Poisson, S., Jolivet, J., Poisson, R., Beretta-Piccoli, M. and Band, R.R. (1979) Tamoxifen induced tumour stimulation and withdrawal response. *Cancer Treat. Rep.*, **63**, 1839–41.

Rosier, J.G. and Underwood, P.B. (1974) Use of progestational agents in endometrial adenocarcinoma. *Obstet. Gynecol.*, **44**, 60–64.

Schiff, I., Sela, H. Km., Cramer, D., Tulchinsky, D. and Ryan, K.J. (1982) Endometrial hyperplasia in women on cyclic or continuous estrogen regimens. *Fertil. Steril.*, **37**, 79–82.

Weiss, M.I. and Sayvetz, T.A. (1980) Incidence of endometrial cancer in relation to the use of oral contraceptives. *New Eng. J. Med.*, **302**, 551–4.

Whitehead, M.I., McQueen, J., Beard, R.J., Minardi, J. and Campbell, S. (1977) The effects of cyclical oestrogen therapy and sequential oestrogen/progesterone therapy on the endometrium of post-menopausal women. *Acta Obstet. Gynecol. Scand.*, (suppl.) **65**, 91–101.

Whitehead, M.I., Townsend, P.T., Pryse-Davies, J., Ryder, T., Lane, G., Siddle, N.C. and King, R.J.B. (1982) Effect of various types and dosages of progestogens on the postmenopausal endometrium. *J. Reprod. Med.*, **27**, 539–48.

World Health Organisation Weekly Epidemiological Record (1982) Non-communicable disease surveillance: oral contraceptives and cancer risk. **57**, 281–8.

6 Endometrial changes associated with intrauterine contraceptive devices

Three basic types of intrauterine contraceptive device (IUCD) are currently encountered, the inert plastic device, which is rarely used nowadays but may still be found in women who have been wearing a device for many years, copper-coated plastic devices, which are in current vogue, and, less commonly, progestagen-impregnated devices. About 50 per cent of women wearing an IUCD have no symptoms attributable to the presence of the device but others may have intermenstrual spotting, menorrhagia, uterine colic or dysmenorrhoea, symptoms which tend to diminish when the device has been in place for some time (Tindall, 1987). A small proportion of women using a device complain of symptoms such as irregular bleeding associated with pelvic pain and vaginal discharge, which suggest a complicating uterine infection. Endometrial biopsy in IUCD wearers may, therefore, be undertaken for the investigation of symptoms secondary to IUCD usage, to confirm or refute the presence of an endometritis or for reasons not directly related to the IUCD, and to which the presence of the device is incidental.

In endometrial biopsies from women wearing an IUCD the principal problem posed to the pathologist is that of distinguishing between inflammatory changes due solely to the mechanical and irritative effects of the IUCD and those due to a superimposed endometrial infection. The local, non-infective, morphological changes induced by an IUCD are largely confined to the superficial layer of the functionalis and are, indeed, localized to the areas of contact between the superficial endometrium and the device. By contrast, changes due to infection are more widespread and extend more deeply into the tissues. If therefore an endometrial biopsy sample contains only tissue from the superficial part of the endometrium it may be possible to assess the direct local effects of the device but impossible to give a histological opinion as to whether or not there is a complicating endometrial infection (Buckley, 1987).

6.1   Local mechanical and irritative changes

Local changes are limited to the contact site of the device and to some extent it is a matter of chance whether this site is included in the biopsy. In the absence of tissue from the contact site a biopsy may show no histological evidence of the presence of an IUCD. It should be noted also that the changes at the contact site are least easily assessed during the late secretory and premenstrual phases of the cycle when they may be masked by the normal physiological changes in the endometrium.

The local pressure of an inert device produces a smooth-contoured depression (Figure 6.1) whilst the copper wire on the stem of a copper-covered device may leave an accurate imprint on the endometrial surface (Figure 6.2) with the formation of a fine papillary pattern, the papillae lying between the coils of the copper wire. The endometrium lying between the device coils or arms may be normal but it is sometimes thrown into oedematous folds, particularly during the early secretory phase (Figure 6.3). In some endometria these folds form polypoidal projections with focally congested and inflamed tips. The surface epithelium at the contact site may be flattened but is not uncommonly

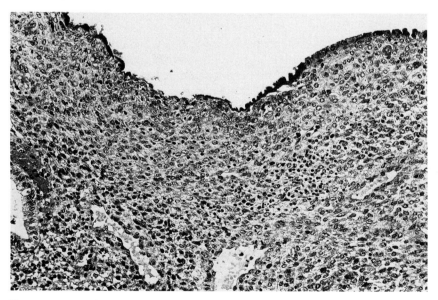

Figure 6.1   Inert intrauterine contraceptive device contact site. The surface of the endometrium is depressed, the epithelium flattened and the underlying stroma pseudodecidualized and infiltrated by a round cell population. Haematoxylin and Eosin × 186.

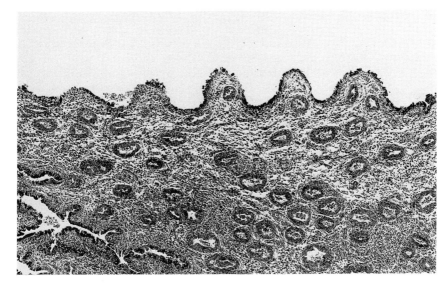

Figure 6.2 Copper-covered intrauterine contraceptive device contact site. The regular indentations created by the copper wire on the shaft of the device are clearly seen. Note that in this case there is little or no underlying inflammation. Haematoxylin and Eosin × 47.

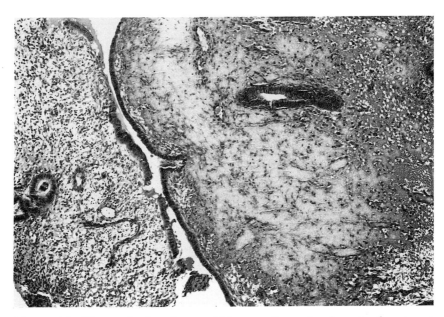

Figure 6.3 The marked oedema which sometimes develops in the stroma between the contact sites of an IUCD is seen in the fragment of endometrium to the right; the endometrium on the left is of more normal appearance. Haematoxylin and Eosin × 93.

absent, having been stripped away by the removal of the device prior to the taking of the biopsy. Beneath some devices there can, however, be true ulceration with the formation of non-specific granulation tissue (Figure 6.4). The epithelium at the margins of an ulcerated contact site may show evidence of regrowth, with mitotic activity and non-specific reactive changes such as nuclear enlargement, nuclear pleomorphism and an increased nucleo-cytoplasmic ratio (Figure 6.5). On rare occasions, when the device has been worn for many years, there can be focal squamous metaplasia at the contact site.

The endometrium immediately below the device is sometimes extremely atrophic and represented by only a thin wisp of stroma, occasionally fibrotic, lacking any glands (Figure 6.4). More commonly the subjacent stroma shows foci of superficial or, less commonly, deep pseudodecidualization (Figure 6.6). Such foci may, in an otherwise unremarkable endometrium, be a clue to the presence of an IUCD. On occasions the endometrial glands immediately deep to the contact site show a pattern of maturation which differs slightly from that in the adjacent areas; the glands may, for instance, show delayed maturation, premature secretory maturation or can, rarely, be inactive.

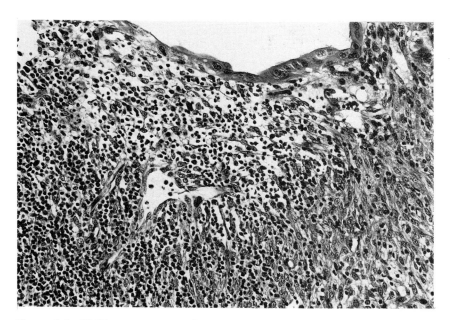

Figure 6.4 IUCD contact site. A flattened surface epithelium lies over a stroma that is devoid of glands, infiltrated by chronic inflammatory cells and partly replaced by maturing non-specific granulation tissue. Haematoxylin and Eosin × 186.

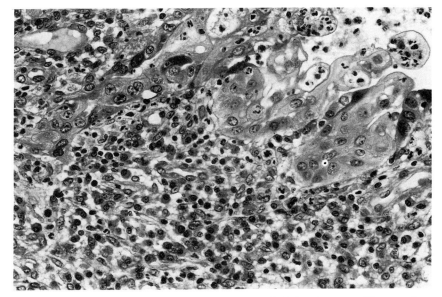

Figure 6.5 IUCD contact site, reactive epithelial changes. The surface epithelium, to the upper right, is formed by cells which vary in shape and size, have lost their polarity and are moderately pleomorphic. The underlying stroma is heavily infiltrated by plasma cells and lymphocytes and the epithelium contains polymorphonuclear leucocytes. Haematoxylin and Eosin × 370.

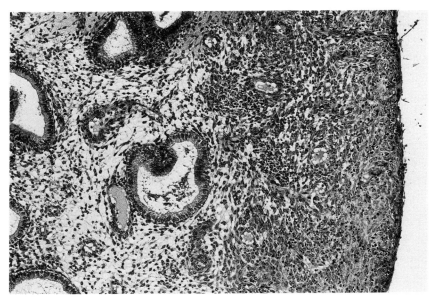

Figure 6.6 Pseudodecidualization of the superficial part of the endometrial stroma (to the right) beneath the contact site of an IUCD. A focal inflammatory infiltrate is also present. Haematoxylin and Eosin × 117.

At the contact site it is usual to find a few polymorphonuclear leucocytes in the surface epithelium (Figure 6.7) together with a focal, mild, non-specific chronic inflammatory cell infiltrate in the subjacent stroma. This infiltrate occasionally forms a sharply defined focus (Figure 6.8) within which the glands may contain occasional polymorphonuclear leucocytes together with nuclear debris. This appearance cannot always be distinguished from early tuberculosis (Chapter 7) but the presence of the other features of a contact site should serve to negate this diagnosis. A foreign body response to an IUCD is distinctly unusual but, occasionally, intraglandular macrophage giant cells are seen (Fox and Buckley, 1983) whilst foreign body granulomas may form around fragments of debris which have become detached from the surface of the device. These are small, associated with minimal local damage and can be in either the deep or superficial layers of the endometrium.

In women wearing a progestagen-impregnated device there are, in addition to the local irritative effects described above, changes attributable to the progestagen. The appearances are similar regardless of

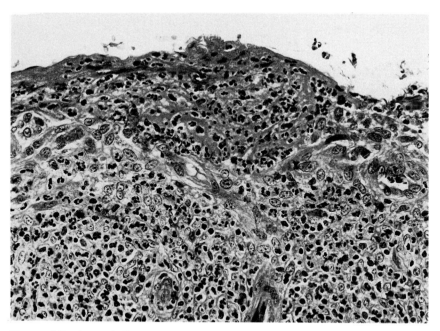

Figure 6.7   Acute inflammation at the contact site of an IUCD. The surface epithelium is intact but shows marked reactive changes and is covered by a layer of acute fibrinous exudate containing numerous polymorphonuclear leucocytes. The underlying stroma is also inflamed. Haematoxylin and Eosin × 370.

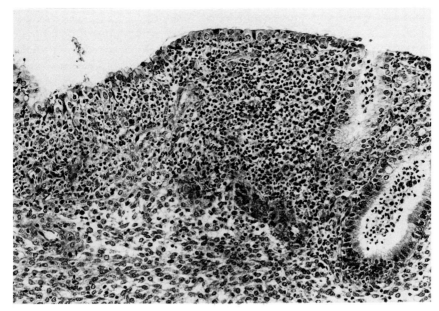

Figure 6.8   A well-demarcated, discrete inflammatory focus at the contact site of an IUCD. In this example the inflammatory infiltrate is composed predominantly of lymphocytes and plasma cells. Haematoxylin and Eosin × 186.

the phase of the menstrual cycle, the duration of IUCD use or the type of progestagen-containing device (Silverberg *et al.*, 1986). Stromal pseudo-decidualization, which is usually most marked in the first months after insertion, and glandular atrophy are typical. Stromal calcification, small polyps and thick-walled fibrotic blood vessels, similar to those seen in endometrial polyps, may develop after several years of use. Rarely, cells with slight nuclear atypia, resembling those in the Arias-Stella phenomenon, are seen in glands lined by otherwise inactive cells.

It should always be borne in mind, when interpreting decidual changes in the endometria of IUCD wearers, that on occasion an intrauterine or ectopic gestation may have occurred and that the decidual change may be indicative of pregnancy. A gestation in one horn of a bicornuate uterus in which the contralateral horn contained an IUCD has also been reported (Tindall, 1987).

6.2   Endometrial infection in IUCD wearers

Some women wearing an IUCD develop a true infective endometritis, probably due to ascending organisms, although this is becoming less common with the change from inert plastic devices to those covered with copper. Infection results in a diffuse endometrial inflammation superimposed on the local inflammatory response evoked by the device acting as an irritative foreign body. Recognition of a complicating endometrial infection depends, therefore, upon the finding of an inflammatory cell infiltrate which extends beyond the contact site. To establish this diagnosis in a biopsy specimen requires, therefore, that endometrial fragments must be sought for which, whilst inflamed, show no evidence of being part of the contact site, a task which is not always easy and is sometimes impossible.

In relatively mild cases of endometrial infection the salient feature is the presence of aggregates of polymorphonuclear leucocytes within, and entirely limited to, glandular lumens over large areas of the endometrium (Figure 6.9). It is unusual for every gland to be affected and, indeed, it is more common to find some variation both in the number of glands affected in a given area and in the degree of involvement. There is usually little or no disturbance of endometrial cyclical maturation with inflammation of this severity and the appearances may suggest a diagnosis of early tuberculosis (Chapter 7).

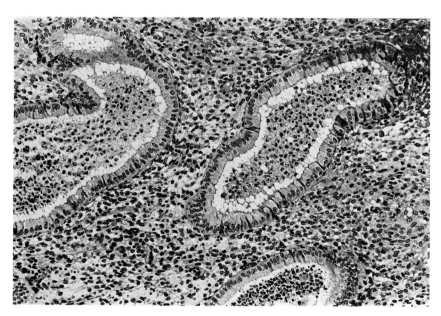

Figure 6.9   Infection of the uterine cavity in an IUCD user. The glands, which are in the mid secretory phase, are filled by a polymorphonuclear leucocyte exudate. Haematoxylin and Eosin × 186.

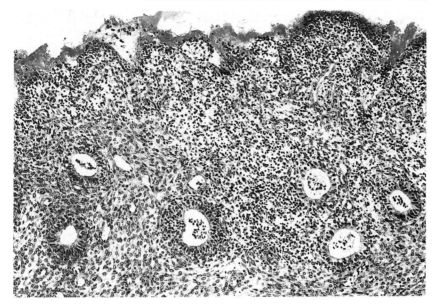

Figure 6.10   Severe non-specific, chronic inflammation in the endometrium of an IUCD user. A predominantly round cell population infiltrates the stroma and the epithelium of the glands. Haematoxylin and Eosin × 117.

A distinction from tuberculosis is usually possible if all the other IUCD related changes in the endometrial biopsy are taken into account but in occasional cases of real doubt it may prove necessary to suggest bacteriological cultures.

With more severe infections the intraglandular polymorphonuclear leucocyte exudate in areas away from the contact site is associated with a diffuse lymphoplasmacytic infiltrate of the stroma (Figure 6.10), the plasma cell component of which is sometimes concentrated around the glands. Infections of this severity tend to inhibit hormone receptor synthesis and hence normal cyclical endometrial maturation is usually disturbed (Figure 6.11). Marked reactive cytological atypia is also a feature commonly found in severe infections (Figure 7.2), whilst biopsies from these patients may also include fragments of heavily inflamed myometrium.

Most endometrial infections complicating IUCD usage are poly-microbial in nature and the inflammatory changes evoked are entirely non-specific. In rare instances, however, an actinomycotic infection occurs, a condition associated with a significant risk of pelvic infection and portal pyaemia (Schiffer *et al.*, 1975; Lomax *et al.*, 1976; Witwer

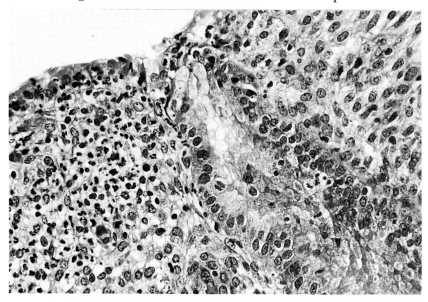

Figure 6.11   Severe, non-specific, chronic inflammation in the endometrium of an IUCD wearer, 24th day of the cycle in a woman with a regular 28 day cycle. Secretory changes are absent and mitotic activity is present in the glandular epithelium. Haematoxylin and Eosin × 370.

et al., 1977; Schmidt *et al.*, 1980). The organisms may be identified in the superficial layers of the endometrium and are accompanied by a polymorphonuclear leucocyte infiltrate. The colonies (sulphur granules) form stellate basophilic structures in haematoxylin and eosin stained sections, and on Gram stains the peripheral margins of the colony are Gram negative whilst the colony is Gram positive.

Correct identification of Actinomyces in an endometrial biopsy is important and can present difficulties for the typical appearances may be mimicked by other intrauterine organisms and by debris (Luff *et al.*, 1978; Jones *et al.*, 1979; Duguid *et al.*, 1980). It is, in fact, only possible to make an accurate diagnosis of Actinomyces if culture or immunohistochemical techniques are employed (Spence *et al.*, 1978; Fry *et al.*, 1980). However, even if the presence of Actinomyces is proven a diagnosis of actinomycotic endometritis is not justified unless there is a definite tissue response to the organism, which can be present as only a commensal. A further factor complicating the diagnosis of actinomycosis in IUCD users is the presence of 'pseudo-sulphur granules' (O'Brien *et al.*, 1981). These are fragments of debris from the surface of the device which form

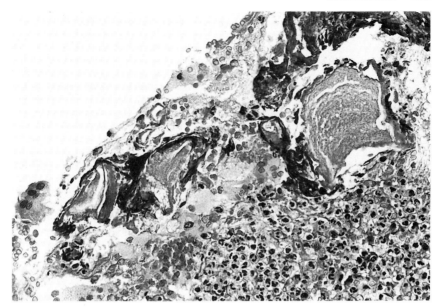

Figure 6.12   The debris from the surface of an intrauterine contraceptive device as it appears in an endometrial curetting: the so-called 'pseudo-sulphur' granules. These may bear a resemblance to bacterial colonies. Haematoxylin and Eosin × 370.

amorphous eosinophilic or basophilic aggregates that bear some resemblance to the sulphur granules found in actinomycotic abscesses (Figure 6.12). Careful histological examination and the employment of a Gram stain usually reveal the true nature of this material.

References

Buckley, C.H. (1987) Pathology of contraception and of hormonal therapy. In *Haines and Taylor: Obstetrical and Gynaecological Pathology* (ed. H. Fox), Churchill Livingstone, Edinburgh, pp. 839–73.

Duguid, H.L., Parratt, D. and Traynor, R. (1980) Actinomyces-like organisms in cervical smears from women using intrauterine contraceptive devices. *Brit. Med. J.*, **281**, 534–7.

Fox, H. and Buckley, C.H. (1983) *Atlas of Gynaecological Pathology*, M.T.P. Press, Lancaster, pp. 159–62.

Fry, R., Linder, A.M. and Bull, M.M. (1980) Actinomyces-like organisms in cervicovaginal smears. *S. Afr. Med. J.*, **57**, 1041–3.

Jones, M.C., Buschmann, B.D., Dowling, E.A. and Pollock, H.M. (1979) The prevalence of actinomycetes-like organisms found in cervico-vaginal smears of 300 IUD wearers. *Acta Cytol.*, **23**, 282–6.

Lomax, C.W., Harbert, E.M. Jr. and Thornton, W.N. Jr. (1976) Actinomycosis of the female genital tract. *Obstet. Gynecol.*, **48**, 341–6.

Luff, R.D., Gupta, P.K., Spence, M.R. and Frost, J.K. (1978) Pelvic actinomycosis and the intra-uterine contraceptive device: a cytohistomorphologic study. *Am. J. Clin. Path.*, **69**, 581–6.

O'Brien, P.K., Roth-Moyo, L.A. and Davis, B.A. (1981) Pseudo-sulfur granules associated with intrauterine contraceptive devices. *Am. J. Clin. Path.*, **75**, 822–5.

Schiffer, M.A., Elguezabal, A., Sultana, M. and Allen, A.C. (1975) Actinomycosis infections associated with intrauterine contraceptive devices. *Obstet. Gynecol.*, **45**, 67–72.

Schmidt, W.A., Bedrossian, C.W.M., Ali, V., Webb, J.A. and Bastian, F.O. (1980) Actinomycosis and intrauterine contraceptive devices: the clinicopathologic entity. *Diag. Gynecol. Obstet.*, **2**, 165–77.

Silverberg, S.G., Haukkamaa, M., Arko, H., Nilsson, C.G. and Luukkainen, T. (1986) Endometrial morphology during long-term use of Levonorgestrel-releasing intrauterine devices. *Int. J. Gynec. Pathol.*, **5**, 235–41.

Spence, M.R., Gupta, P.K., Frost, J.K. and King, T.M. (1978) Cytologic detection and clinical significance of *Actinomyces israelii* in women using intrauterine contraceptive devices. *Am. J. Obstet. Gynecol.*, **131**, 295–8.

Tindall, V.R. (1987) *Jeffcoate's Principles of Gynaecology*, Butterworths, London, pp. 608.

Witwer, M.W., Farmer, M.F., Wand, J.S. and Solomon, L.S. (1977) Extensive actinomycosis associated with an intrauterine contraceptive device. *Am. J. Obstet. Gynecol.*, **128**, 913–14.

7 Inflammation of the endometrium

Endometrial inflammation may be of infective or non-infective origin and is recognized histologically by the identification of an abnormal pattern of inflammatory cell infiltrate and by disturbances in the normal processes of endometrial growth and maturation. The diagnosis of endometritis depends entirely upon such histopathological criteria because the clinical correlates of endometrial inflammation are both variable and inconsistent.

The diagnosis of an endometritis is complicated by the fact that many of the features which, in other tissues, indicate the presence of an inflammatory process are found in the normal endometrium. Thus, for example, a polymorphonuclear leucocytic infiltrate, interstitial haemorrhage and tissue necrosis accompany menstruation or hormone withdrawal bleeding whilst tissue regeneration occurs not only following inflammation but also in the immediate postmenstrual phase. Furthermore, lymphocytes, lymphoid aggregates and lymphoid follicles with germinal centres which, in association with macrophages, are regarded elsewhere in the body as indicators of chronic inflammation all occur in the normal endometrium (Payan et al, 1964; Sen and Fox, 1967). Other more precise criteria are therefore needed for the diagnosis of inflammation in the endometrium and paramount among these are the finding of plasma cells and eosinophils, both of which are absent from the normal endometrium (Hendrickson and Kempson, 1980).

The reported incidence of chronic endometritis ranges from 2.8% (Vasudeva et al., 1972) to 19.2% (Farooki, 1967) in series which include biopsy, curettage and hysterectomy specimens and samples from non-pregnant, post-abortive and postpartum patients.

Excluding post-abortive and postpartum material, the incidence in our practice of active, chronic endometritis is 3.08% in biopsy material which is much lower than the 10.86% recorded for hysterectomy specimens in the same hospital. This suggests that there may be a sampling error when only small biopsies are examined or, alternatively, that superficial

105

specimens fail to detect inflammation in the deeper parts of the functionalis or in the basalis (Kitching, 1984).

Cases of endometrial inflammation are usually classified into those in which the pathological features are non-specific and those in which the findings are sufficiently typical as to suggest a specific aetiological factor.

7.1   Non-specific endometritis

The term 'non-specific endometritis' refers to the presence within the endometrium of a range of inflammatory changes which offer little or no clue to their cause. It is, however, customary to distinguish pathologically between the acute and chronic phases of the disorder and between infective and non-infective causes, although the clinical correlates are rarely so clearly defined and in practice, in the absence of microbiological studies, it is impossible to distinguish infective from non-infective endometritis. Further, many conditions in which the cause may initially be non-infective, such as the inflammation which accompanies tissue breakdown, may, if they persist, predispose to the establishment of non-specific infection. The distinction between the acute and chronic phases may also become blurred as the two often have a common origin and similar clinico-pathological correlates (Buckley, 1987).

7.1.1   The aetiology and clinical correlates of non-specific endometritis

Non-specific endometrial inflammation occurs under a variety of conditions many of which have in common one or more of the following factors: disruption of the cervical mucous barrier, intrauterine stasis or necrosis, interruption of regular endometrial shedding or hindrance to natural drainage. Disruption of the cervical mucous barrier occurs when an organism has the capacity to penetrate the mucus, when there is cervical infection or surgery (Rotterdam, 1978; Greenwood and Moran, 1981) or when the tail of an IUCD protrudes through the external os (Chapter 6). Intrauterine necrosis may occur under a wide variety of circumstances, for example on the tip of a polyp or sub-mucous leiomyoma, during spontaneous abortion, around an IUCD, in the post-abortive or postpartum state, in patients with an intrauterine neoplasm (where it may also be part of an immunological response) and in women with dysfunctional uterine haemorrhage. Intrauterine stasis may also occur in many of the preceding circumstances but more typically results from stenosis of the cervix or distortion of the cavity by a space-occupying lesion.

Pregnancy may be associated with an acute or chronic inflammatory cell infiltrate (see below) and following radiotherapy to the genital tract a non-specific or, less commonly, a granulomatous inflammation may occur.

In patients with acute endometritis there is commonly an immediately recognizable predisposing factor such as pregnancy, abortion, parturition or a recent surgical procedure to the cervix or uterine body. In patients with chronic inflammation of the endometrium, by contrast, there are rarely any identifiable causes and the patient can be asymptomatic or may present with abnormal uterine bleeding, abdominal pain, infertility or vaginal discharge.

7.1.2   The diagnosis of non-specific endometritis

The morphological response of the endometrium to inflammatory agents is of limited range and strictly speaking a diagnosis of infection should be made only when both an infecting organism and a morphological response can be identified. However, in practice, microbiological studies are not always performed and the finding of an inflammatory process in the endometrium should always rouse the suspicion that it may be of an infective origin.

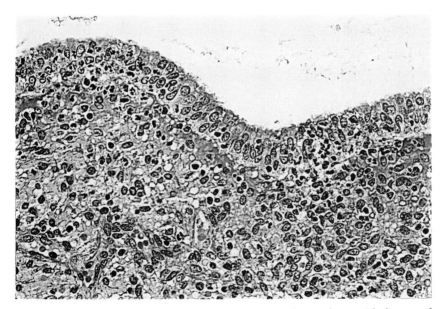

Figure 7.1 Mild acute, non-specific endometritis. The surface epithelium and underlying stroma contain a scanty infiltrate of polymorphonuclear leucocytes; the aetiology in this case was unknown. Haematoxylin and Eosin × 370.

Mild acute inflammation (Figure 7.1) is often limited to the superficial layers of the endometrium and is recognized by the presence of a polymorphonuclear leucocytic infiltrate within the glands and in the endometrial stroma. There may be a minor degree of stromal necrosis together with epithelial disruption on the endometrial surface and in the superficial parts of the glands. Inflammation of this degree can occur at any stage of the endometrial cycle, and in the non-cycling endometrium, and may be diffuse and widespread or focal and local. It must be distinguished from the physiological infiltrate of normal menstruation and the scanty, multifocal aggregates of polymorphonuclear leucocytes which are a normal concomitant of decidual remodelling in early pregnancy.

When the inflammatory process is severe, the infiltrate extends through the full thickness of the endometrium to involve the basalis. There is almost invariably a non-specific reactive change in the endometrial epithelium, characterized by variation in cell size, nuclear

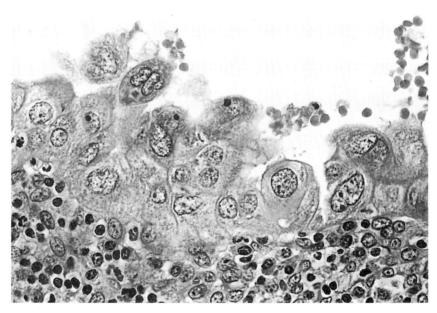

Figure 7.2 Pyometra. The surface epithelium of the endometrium in a 72 year old woman who had a pyometra with utero-colonic fistula associated with diverticular disease of the large bowel. The epithelial cells are enlarged, the nuclei are pleomorphic and have lost their polarity. One nucleus contains a nucleolus; one cell is binucleate and nuclear chromatin is coarse. Haematoxylin and Eosin × 594.

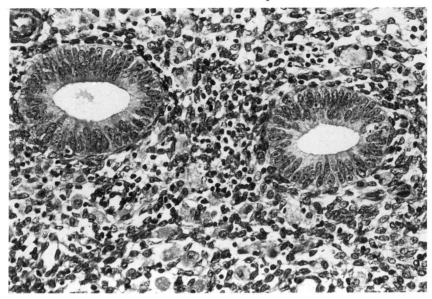

Figure 7.3 Non-specific chronic endometritis. The basalis of a patient who presented with secondary infertility. The stroma is heavily infiltrated by histiocytes and lymphocytes. A similar appearance is sometimes seen in women with polymenorrhoea. Haematoxylin and Eosin × 370.

enlargement and pleomorphism, formation of nucleoli and mitotic activity (Figure 7.2). The more severe the inflammation, the more likely it is to disturb the normal process of endometrial maturation although this is a common feature of the chronically inflamed endometrium (see below).

Chronic non-granulomatous inflammation of the endometrium (Figure 7.3) is recognized by those features which in other tissues also constitute the hallmarks of chronic inflammation, these being the presence of a cellular infiltrate containing plasma cells, lymphocytes, macrophages (which may contain haemosiderin), occasional polymorphonuclear leucocytes and eosinophils. In the active chronic phase (Figure 7.4) it is usual to identify polymorphonuclear leucocytes and plasma cells and, in some instances, the pattern may be characterized by an accumulation of polymorphonuclear leucocytes in the glands and a plasma cell infiltrate which is concentrated in the periglandular stroma (Figure 7.5). Sometimes there is a conspicuous infiltrate in the superficial layers of the functionalis (Figure 7.6). More commonly, however, even in moderately severe; active chronic inflammation, plasma cells are relatively few in

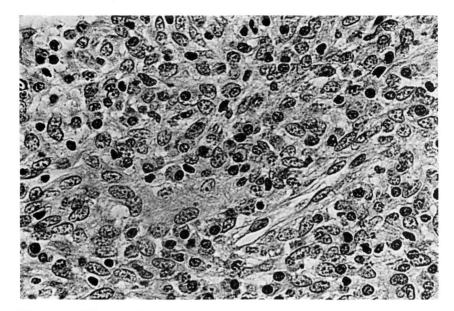

Figure 7.4 Non-specific active chronic endometritis, three months post partum, in a patient with irregular and excessive bleeding. The stroma is heavily infiltrated by plasma cells and occasional lymphocytes. An inflammatory infiltrate so long after delivery is abnormal. Haematoxylin and Eosin × 594.

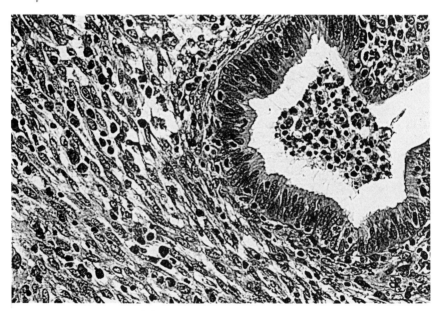

Figure 7.5 Non-specific endometritis. The inflammatory infiltrate is characterized by stromal plasma cells and lymphocytes and intraglandular polymorphonuclear leucocytes and histiocytes. Haematoxylin and Eosin × 370.

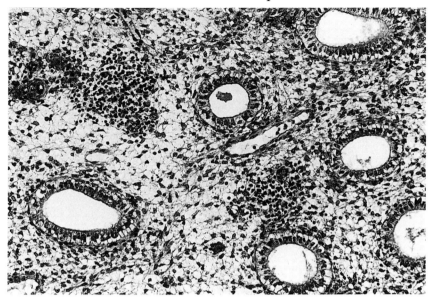

Figure 7.6 Non-specific active chronic endometritis. Aggregates of lymphocytes and plasma cells in the functionalis of an endometrium from a patient whose intrauterine contraceptive device had been removed, because of pelvic pain and vaginal discharge, 17 days previously. Haematoxylin and Eosin × 186.

number; they are most easily identified in the endometrium at the junction of the basalis and functionalis and may therefore be overlooked in a superficial biopsy. In the puerperium, a similar infiltrate of plasma cells, lymphocytes and macrophages can be regarded as physiological (Hendrickson and Kempson, 1980) although its persistence beyond the fourth week of the puerperium is abnormal and usually associated with persistent bleeding, retained products of conception or infection. The endometrium of a woman with perimenopausal bleeding also often contains a non-specific inflammatory cell infiltrate and in such cases the inflammation may be the consequence of the repeated or persistent breakdown of tissue rather than its cause.

In a less active chronic endometritis, the inflammatory cell infiltrate may be almost entirely lymphocytic (Figure 7.7) and it is this form which is most difficult both to identify and to differentiate from the normal lymphocytic complement. Indeed, many regard the presence of eosinophils or plasma cells as a prerequisite for the diagnosis of chronic endometritis (Brudenell, 1955; Cadena *et al.*, 1973); and will not entertain this diagnosis in their absence. In this respect the use of

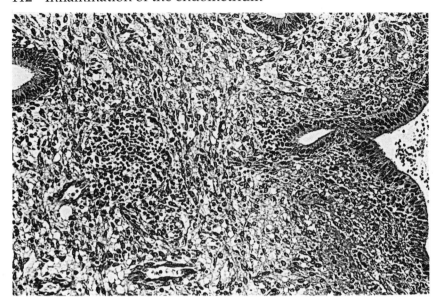

Figure 7.7 Chronic non-specific endometritis. Lymphocytic aggregates in the functionalis in an asymptomatic patient. The biopsy was taken routinely prior to sterilization. Haematoxylin and Eosin × 186.

immunohistochemical techniques (Crum *et al.*, 1983) for the identification of immunoglobulins may prove helpful in the recognition of small numbers of plasma cells, particularly if the tissues are first trypsinized. Others have found Unna Pappenheim stained sections useful for the same purpose (Horton and Wilkes, 1976). Certainly a diagnosis based upon the recognition of an increased number of lymphocytes and the occurrence of more than the usual number of lymphoid aggregates or lymphoid follicles is often more subjective than objective, and genuine cases of chronic inflammation are undoubtedly overlooked in the anxiety not to succumb to overdiagnosis. We would regard as suspicious those cases in which the lymphoid aggregates or follicles occur in the functional layers of the endometrium or when patchy lymphocytic infiltrates are present (Figure 7.8).

A dense chronic inflammation has to be distinguished from the monotonous infiltrate of a leukaemia or lymphoma and from an endometrial stromal sarcoma (Chapters 11 and 12).

Fibrosis and the formation of non-specific granulation tissue are distinctly uncommon in the endometrium, even in long-established disease (Hendrickson and Kempson, 1980) but may sometimes be found

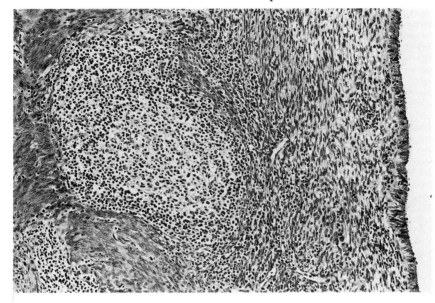

Figure 7.8 Chronic non-specific endometritis. Lymphoid follicles are seen in the basalis and superficial myometrium in a hysterectomy specimen. There was cervical stenosis and the patient had had a pyometra which had been treated by antibiotics for several weeks prior to surgery. Haematoxylin and Eosin × 149.

when an IUCD is present (Figure 6.4) or when there has been a particularly destructive inflammation. The possibility that non-specific granulation tissue in an endometrial biopsy may, in fact, have come from the cervix should always be considered.

In both severe acute and chronic inflammation the endometrium is often poorly developed. It is shallow, the glands are tubular and inactive, or only weakly proliferative, and their lining epithelium may show severe, non-specific reactive changes. The cells become stratified, tend to have an increased nucleo-cytoplasmic ratio and may show some loss of nuclear polarity with nuclear pleomorphism and the formation of nucleoli. Cytoplasmic vacuolation may be prominent, and indeed the atypia of these cells can be so marked as to mimic a neoplastic process. The stroma may be unusually compact and have a rather fibrotic appearance (Figure 7.9) whilst the stromal cells often palisade around the glands to create a 'pinwheel' effect (Kurman, 1982). The poor or negligible response to hormonal stimulation which occurs in the severely inflamed endometrium is the consequence of a failure of hormone receptor formation. It is difficult or impossible, therefore, in these samples to assess the patient's hormonal status.

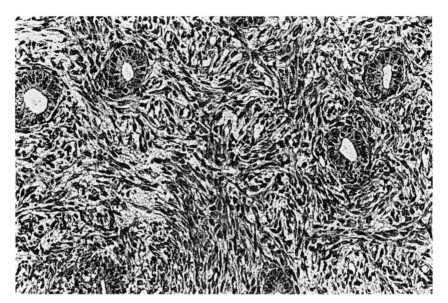

Figure 7.9 Non-specific chronic endometritis. This endometrium, from a patient who had worn an inert intrauterine contraceptive device, has a rather fibrous stroma in which there is a scanty lymphocytic infiltrate. The glands are poorly responsive. Haematoxylin and Eosin × 186.

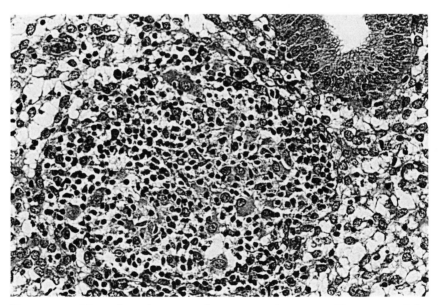

Figure 7.10 Non-tuberculous granulomatous endometritis. The centre of the field is occupied by a well-formed foreign body type granuloma. Microbiological studies were negative and no foreign material was identified. The cause remains a mystery. Haematoxylin and Eosin × 370.

We have only rarely encountered non-specific granulomatous endometritis, usually in the presence of an IUCD, following radiotherapy for carcinoma of the cervix or in response to keratin from metaplastic squamous foci or squamous carcinoma. The granulomas tend to be very poorly formed and consist of no more than an aggregate of macrophages or foreign body giant cells (Figure 7.10).

7.1.2   Morphologically distinct forms of non-specific chronic endometritis

(a) *Histiocytic endometritis*   The end stage of a pyometra or haematometra may be recognized by the presence of a histiocytic endometritis (Buckley and Fox, 1980), a lesion also known as xanthogranulomatous endometritis. The endometrium is replaced or heavily infiltrated by foamy lipid-containing histiocytes intermingled with macrophage giant cells (in which there may be cholesterol clefts), plasma cells, lymphocytes and occasional polymorphonuclear leucocytes (Figure 7.11). The histiocytes stain positively with Sudan Black and Oil Red-O and are also PAS, diastase resistant, positive. The content of

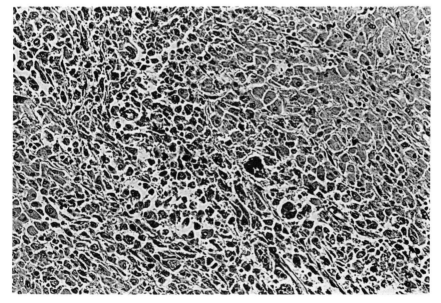

Figure 7.11   Histiocytic (xanthogranulomatous) endometritis. The endometrium is almost entirely replaced by sheets of histiocytes, many of which contain haemosiderin. A lymphocytic infiltrate is also present. In this case, the condition represents the end stage of a haematometra. Haematoxylin and Eosin × 232.

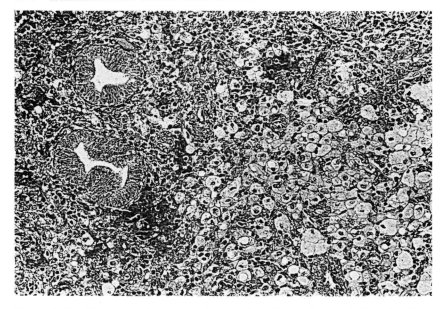

Figure 7.12   Chronic endometritis characterized by histiocytic infiltration. The specimen was taken six weeks postpartum from a woman who complained of continued bleeding. Note that the glands (to the left) show no evidence of cyclical changes. Haematoxylin and Eosin × 186.

haemosiderin in the histiocytes is variable and dependent upon the degree of preceding haemorrhage. The absence of Michaelis–Gutmann bodies distinguishes the condition from malakoplakia. A similar, though less intense, histiocytic infiltrate is seen in a wide variety of other conditions such as the post-abortive or post-delivery endometrium (Figure 7.12) or in association with chronic cervical stenosis, endometrial hyperplasia or carcinoma (Figure 10.4).

(b) *Malakoplakia*   Malakoplakia is a histological expression of an abnormal immunological response to bacteria. The histological appearances of endometrial malakoplakia are similar to those of histiocytic endometritis. The stroma of the endometrium is heavily infiltrated, and may be entirely replaced over large areas by sheets of foamy histiocytes (von Hansemann's histiocytes) which differ in appearance from those seen in histiocytic endometritis only by the presence of Michaelis–Gutmann bodies (Figure 7.13). These are small, round laminated calcipherites which are found not only in the cytoplasm of the histiocytes but also extracellularly. They contain calcium which can be identified using von Kossa's stain; they are also PAS positive and

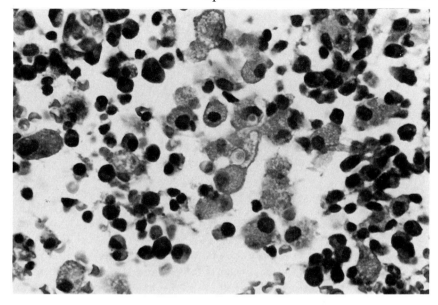

Figure 7.13 Malakoplakia. The specimen consists almost entirely of histiocytes, lymphocytes and plasma cells. In the centre of the field, there are several histiocytes in which spherical intracytoplasmic inclusions, Michaelis-Gutmann bodies, can be seen. Haematoxylin and Eosin × 743.

contain lysozyme (Molnar and Poliak, 1983). A mixed inflammatory infiltrate of plasma cells, polymorphonuclear leucocytes and lymphocytes is usually mixed with the histiocytes.

Admixed bacteria, most commonly *E. coli*, which are retained within the phagolysosomes of the macrophages are not digested and can be identified at light and electron microscopic levels in the cytoplasm of the histiocytes and in extracellular sites.

Clinically, malakoplakia is a rare cause of postmenopausal bleeding (Thomas *et al.*, 1978; Molnar and Poliak, 1983).

7.2 Specific forms of endometritis

7.2.1 *Viral infections*

(*a*) *Herpes virus hominis*   Herpetic endometritis is characterized by the presence of enlarged epithelial nuclei with a ground glass appearance, beading of the nuclear membranes and epithelial multinucleation. Eosinophilic intranuclear viral inclusions with clear haloes can be seen in both stromal and epithelial cells in haematoxylin and eosin stained sections (Abraham, 1978; Schneider *et al.*, 1982) and their presence is confirmed by either electron microscopy or immunohistochemical techniques. There may also be endometrial necrosis and a lymphocytic infiltrate. In the absence of virological investigations, difficulties have been reported in distinguishing intranuclear pseudoinclusions in a patient with Arias-Stella change from those due to herpes (Dardi *et al.*, 1982).

Infection of the endometrium occurs in association with herpetic infection of the cervix, vagina and vulva (Goldman, 1970) and immuno-suppression may predispose to its development.

(*b*) *Cytomegalovirus* Cytomegalovirus infection of the endometrium is rare (Weller, 1971; Dehner and Askin, 1975) and is characterized by a diffuse lymphoplasmacytic infiltrate in which there are occasional eosinophils (McCracken *et al.*, 1974) and lymphoid follicles with poorly-formed germinal centres (Wenkebach and Curry, 1976). In the nuclei of both stromal and glandular epithelial cells there are large amphophilic to basophilic inclusions measuring 20 to 25 μm in diameter; these are separated from the nuclear membrane by a clear space traversed by fine chromatin strands (Dehner and Askin, 1975). The same cells also contain small, basophilic, P.A.S. positive cytoplasmic inclusions.

An Arias-Stella reaction with marked nuclear enlargement may be confused histologically with cytomegalovirus infection (Kurman, 1982), but the recognition of pregnancy-type hypersecretory endometrium throughout the biopsy specimen should make possible the avoidance of this diagnostic solecism.

7.2.2   Chlamydial infections

The intensity of the inflammatory infiltrate in chlamydial endometritis is variable. In the acute phase there may be a non-specific, polymorphonuclear leucocyte infiltrate of such severity that it suggests a pyogenic infection whilst in the chronic phase the infiltrate is predominantly plasmolymphocytic (Schachter, 1978) and may include lymphoid aggregates and follicles. Stromal necrosis is a common finding and this may be so severe that it mimics menstrual breakdown (Winkler *et al.*, 1984). As with other severe inflammatory processes, reactive atypia of the endometrial epithelium is commonly seen.

Typical *C. trachomatis* inclusion bodies have been demonstrated in the epithelial cells of patients with chlamydial endometritis (Mardh *et al.*, 1981; Ingerslev *et al.*, 1982; Weström, 1982) but these are difficult, if not impossible, to detect with confidence in haematoxylin and eosin stained sections. They can, however, be seen a little more easily in Giemsa stained material and identified specifically using immunohistochemical techniques (Winkler *et al.*, 1984). Using a specific antibody and an immunoperoxidase technique, staining is focal and localized to the epithelial cells where it appears as dark brown stippling within well-circumscribed, rounded, supranuclear, intracytoplasmic vacuoles. These positive areas correspond in haematoxylin and eosin stained sections to intracytoplasmic vacuoles filled with pale staining, faintly basophilic, particles. Positive granules are also seen in mucus, within polymorpho-nuclear leucocytes and on the surface epithelium (Winkler *et al.*, 1984).

Chlamydial infection has been implicated not only as a cause of acute and chronic endometritis but also as a possible aetiological factor in otherwise unexplained infertility (Gump *et al.*, 1981; Mardh *et al.*, 1981; Ingerslev *et al.*, 1982; Wølner-Hanssen *et al.*, 1982). It is a recognized cause of menometrorrhagia, intermenstrual bleeding, pelvic pain and yellow-white vaginal discharge (Gump *et al.*, 1981; Mardh *et al.*, 1981; Winkler *et al.*, 1984).

7.2.3   Bacterial infections

(a)   *Tuberculosis*   This endometrial disease is now rather uncommon in most western countries but still occurs with considerable frequency in many countries of the developing world. Tuberculosis of the endometrium is generally most common in the reproductive years, reaching a peak in the third and fourth decades (Schaefer *et al.*, 1972), though there appears to have been a trend in recent years for the disease to affect a slightly older age group (Hutchins, 1977) with a mean of 42 years. During the reproductive years it is diagnosed most commonly during the investigation of infertility and presents less commonly as amenorrhoea, pelvic pain or heavy and irregular menses (Schaefer, 1970; Bazaz-Malik *et al.*, 1983). After the menopause, tuberculous endometritis is most likely to present as abnormal uterine bleeding in a parous patient (Schaefer *et al.*, 1972).

Infection of the endometrium usually occurs by direct transluminal spread from the Fallopian tube to the superficial layers of the functionalis. Unless ovulation, and hence menstruation, cease, the infected endometrium will be shed monthly, thus allowing only 22 to 23 days for the establishment of infection. It is, therefore, uncommon in endometrial biopsies to see well-established tuberculoid granulomas, which typically take a minimum of 15 days to form (Rotterdam, 1978). Biopsies taken in the premenstrual phase have the greatest chance of providing a positive morphological diagnosis since the granulomas have had the longest time to develop (Figure 7.14). However, despite regular shedding of the endometrium infection is known to affect the basalis in up to 40% of cases

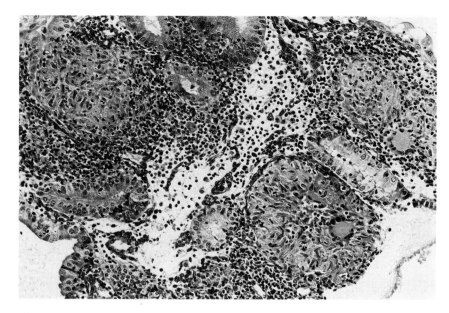

Figure 7.14 Tuberculous endometritis. A curettage sample containing particularly well-developed tuberculous granulomas. Langerhans giant cells are prominent and there is also a marked lymphocytic infiltrate. Haematoxylin and Eosin × 149.

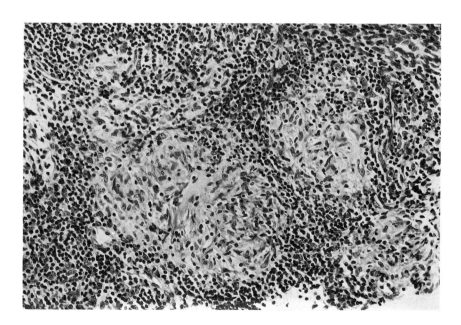

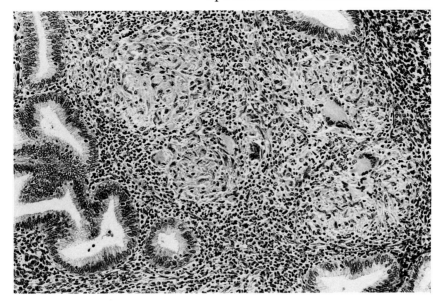

Figure 7.16   Tuberculous endometritis. In the basalis of this sample there are well-formed granulomas. Their presence suggests that shedding of the infected tissue was incomplete in the previous cycle and demonstrates that even in the reproductive years infection is not limited to the functionalis. Haematoxylin and Eosin × 186.

(Nogales-Ortiz *et al.*, 1979) and certainly tuberculosis of the endometrium can develop, probably from this source but possibly from haematogenous spread, even after removal of the Fallopian tubes.

The most typical findings in tuberculosis occur in the regularly menstruating woman. Small, isolated, frequently sparse, ill-formed granulomas are scattered throughout the functionalis. They consist of an aggregate of epithelioid macrophages surrounded by a cuff of lymphocytes (Govan, 1962) and do not often contain giant cells (Figure 7.15). Caseation is rarely observed in these granulomas (Haines and Stallworthy, 1952) except after the menopause, or in the unusual event that the severity of the systemic disease impairs ovulation. Sometimes, however, granulomas in different stages of development co-exist

Figure 7.15   Tuberculous endometritis. The ill-formed granulomas which are more typical of tuberculosis in the endometrium. Epithelioid macrophages form aggregates and have a cuff of lymphocytes but there is no caseation or giant cell formation. Haematoxylin or Eosin × 232.

suggesting that complete shedding of the functionalis has not occurred and that some granulomas have persisted from the previous cycle. These are identified by their morphological maturity and by the more frequent presence of giant cells (Figure 7.16).

Granulomas often lie adjacent to, and bulge into, glands and lymphocytes from their peripheral cuff may infiltrate into the glandular epithelium (Figure 7.17). These individual glands frequently show a lack of secretory response (Nogales-Ortiz et al., 1979). Less commonly there may be a generalized 'poor secretory' pattern (Govan, 1962) in which the endometrium is oedematous and the stromal cells spindle-shaped and lacking in decidual change. The glandular epithelium is cuboidal and has glassy, translucent cytoplasm with well-defined cell borders. Many glands are empty but in some there may be a trace of PAS positive material.

Biopsies taken in the early part of the menstrual cycle may fail to show evidence of granulomatous inflammation and reveal only a non-specific picture of intrastromal plasma cells and lymphocytes or intraglandular polymorphonuclear leucocytes, seen particularly in dilated glands in the deeper part of the functionalis (Govan, 1962) (Figure 7.18). The presence

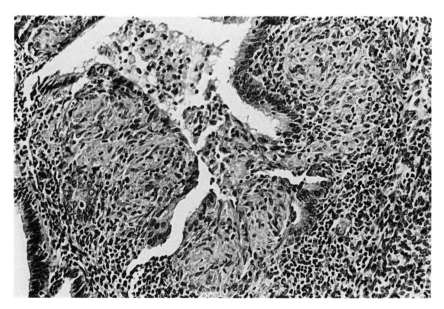

Figure 7.17 Tuberculous endometritis. Granulomas often form on the margins of glands and protrude into their lumens. Glandular epithelium may be disrupted by their presence as in this case. Haematoxylin and Eosin × 232.

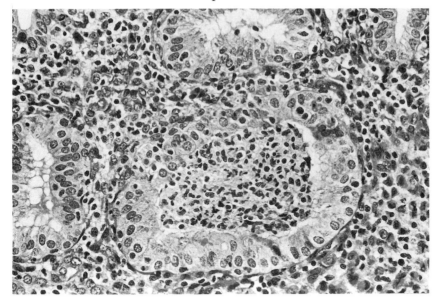

Figure 7.18   Tuberculous endometritis, non-specific appearance. In this area, in the endometrium of a patient with positive cultures for *M. tuberculosis*, there is no evidence of granuloma formation but the gland contains polymorphonuclear leucocytes and the surrounding stroma contains lymphocytes. Haematoxylin and Eosin × 370.

of plasma cells in the endometrium of a woman with tuberculosis may indicate that there is a secondary pyogenic infection (Govan, 1962); clinically this is important as the patient may develop acute symptoms following curettage.

In some cases tuberculous granulomas of the endometrium closely resemble those seen in sarcoidosis, even to the presence of Schauman bodies. However, sarcoidosis has been reported only rarely in the endometrium (Ho, 1979), invariably in women with widespread systemic disease, and as a general working rule all granulomas should initially be regarded as tuberculous in nature until proved otherwise. As acid/alcohol fast bacilli are seldom found in Ziehl-Neelsen stained section of the endometrium confirmatory cultures should be carried out in all cases in which histological examination raises the possibility of tuberculosis.

After the menopause tuberculous endometritis is rare, a fact attributed to the diminished vascularity of the tissue (Schaefer *et al.*, 1972), but when it does occur the infection may become well established because of the absence of regular shedding. The lesions progress to the stage of caseation and biopsy material may consist only of confluent caseating granulomas; there may also be calcification. Residual endometrial glands may show non-specific, reactive changes of the type described in active, non-specific, chronic inflammation (see above).

The differential diagnosis of tuberculosis of the endometrium should include infections due to fungi, schistosomiasis, pinworm infestations, *T. mycoplasma* infection, sarcoidosis, foreign body granulomas, post-irradiation granulomas and granulomas associated with giant cell vasculitis.

(*b*) *Gonorrhoea Neisseria gonorrhoea* is one of the relatively few organisms which have the ability to penetrate the cervical mucous barrier (Moyer, 1975) and can induce an acute, though transient, endometritis.

The superficial layers of the endometrium become heavily infiltrated by polymorphonuclear leucocytes and there is a variable degree of superficial necrosis (Figure 7.19). *N. gonorrhoea* has also been implicated in chronic, non-specific endometritis. It has been our experience that the endometrial damage is limited to the superficial layers and that this

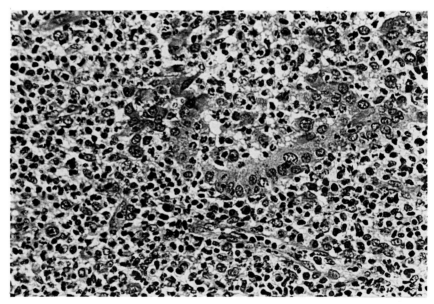

Figure 7.19 Gonococcal endometritis. A severe, necrotizing endometritis from a patient with positive cultures for *N. gonorrhoea*. The gland in the centre of the field contains polymorphonuclear leucocytes and its wall is partly destroyed. The surrounding stroma contains a mixture of plasma cells and lymphocytes. Haematoxylin and Eosin × 370.

finding was quite unexpected in patients who were asymptomatic but in whom nevertheless microbiological studies demonstrated the presence of *N. gonorrhoea*.

(c) *Neisseria meningitidis*   N. *meningitidis* has been isolated from a patient with endometritis-salpingitis-peritonitis (Monif, 1981), although no details were given of the histopathological features of the endometrial infection. In practice, the organism is hard to identify and Gram negative, oxidase-positive diplococci are usually assumed to be gonococci.

(d) *Actinomyces israelii*   Actinomycosis of the endometrium is rare but has been reported in patients wearing an IUCD (Chapter 6).

7.2.4 Mycoplasma hominis

Patients in whom cultures for M. *hominis* are positive have a subtle endometritis with minute, focal collections of lymphocytes, macrophages, occasional polymorphonuclear leucocytes and rare plasma cells (Horne *et al.*, 1973). The infiltrate tends to lie immediately below the endometrial surface epithelium, adjacent to glands or around spiral arteries.

M. *hominis* has been implicated, not always convincingly, as an aetiological factor in infertility, pelvic inflammatory disease (Møller, 1983), postpartum endometritis (Gibbs *et al.*, 1983) and non-specific plasma cell endometritis (Paavonen *et al.*, 1983).

7.2.5 Mycoses

Fungal endometritis is distinctly rare. *Blastomyces dermatidis* (Hamblen *et al.*, 1935; Farber *et al.*, 1968), *Coccidioides immitus* (Saw *et al.*, 1975; Hart *et al.*, 1976) and *Cryptococcus glabratus* (Plaut, 1950) all elicit a granulomatous inflammatory response with epithelioid tubercles which must be distinguished from tuberculosis by using silver stains to demonstrate the fungi. Each organism has distinctive morphological characteristics. *Blastomyces* has a single budding yeast form, *Coccidioides* forms a large spherule in which endospores can be seen and *Cryptococcus* grows as a round or oval budding intracellular or extracellular organism with a thick, mucicarmine positive gelatinous capsule. Sometimes *Cryptococcus* elicits not a granulomatous but a neutrophil polymorphonuclear leucocytic exudative reaction. *Candida* (Rodriguez *et al.*, 1972) tends to grow over the surface of the endometrium and is associated with a plasmalymphocytic infiltrate in the adjacent stroma. It has an oval yeast-like form and produces pseudohyphae which can be demonstrated in histological preparations using a P.A.S. stain or a silver technique such as Gomori methenamine silver.

7.2.6   Protozoan infections

(*a*)   *Toxoplasma gondii*   The inflammatory response to *Toxoplasma gondii* is entirely non-specific. The predominantly extracellular organisms are scattered throughout the endometrial stroma and are difficult to detect with light microscopy. The parasites have been identified in the endometrium and menstrual blood of women with habitual abortion.

(*b*)   *Schistosomiasis*   The presence, in the endometrium, of the ova of *Schistosomiasis haematobium* or, less commonly, *S. mansoni* elicits a granulomatous inflammation. The ova are surrounded by multinucleated macrophage giant cells, epithelioid cells, eosinophils, lymphocytes and plasma cells, with fibroblasts forming a peripheral zone. Frequently, by the time of diagnosis the ova have calcified and the inflammatory response may be mild (Berry, 1966; Williams, 1967) or occasionally so severe that the consequent fibrosis may result in amenorrhoea (Mouktar, 1966).

7.2.7   Miscellaneous parasitic infestations

Other parasitic infections of the endometrium are exceptionally rare. Pinworms (*Enterobius vermicularis*) produce a granulomatous endometritis characterized by the presence of the female worm in the basalis surrounded by successive zones of coagulative necrosis, eosinophils, epithelioid cells, lymphocytes and fibrous tissue (Schenken and Tamisea, 1956).

References

Abraham, A.A. (1978) Herpes virus hominis endometritis in a young woman wearing an intrauterine contraceptive device. *Am. J. Obstet. Gynecol.*, **131**, 340–42.

Bazaz-Malik, G., Maheshwari, B. and Lal, N. (1983) Tuberculous endometritis: a clinico-pathological study of 1000 cases. *Brit. J. Obstet. Gynaecol.*, **90**, 84–6.

Berry, A. (1966) A cytopathological and histopathological study of bilharziasis of the female genital tract. *J. Pathol. Bacteriol.*, **91**, 325–38.

Brudenell, J.M. (1955) Chronic endometritis and plasma cell infiltration of the endometrium. *J. Obstet. Gynaecol. Brit. Emp.*, **62**, 269–74.

Buckley, C.H. (1987) Endometrial inflammation. In *Haines and Taylor: Obstetrical and Gynaecological Pathology* (ed. H. Fox), Churchill Livingstone, Edinburgh, London, pp. 340–53.

Buckley, C.H. and Fox, H. (1980) Histiocytic endometritis. *Histopathology*, **4**, 105–10.

Cadena, D., Cavanzo, F.J., Leone, C.L. and Taylor, H.B. (1973) Chronic endometritis: a comparative clinicopathologic study. *Obstet. Gynecol.*, **41**, 733–8.

Crum, C.P., Egawa, K., Fenoglio, C.M. and Richart, R.M. (1983) Chronic endometritis: the role of immunohistochemistry in the detection of plasma cells. *Am. J. Obstet. Gynecol.* **147**, 812–15.

Dardi, L.E., Ariano, L., Ariano, M.C. and Gould, V.E. (1982) Arias-Stella reaction with prominent nuclear pseudoinclusions simulating herpetic endometritis. *Diag. Gynecol. Obstet.*, **4**, 127–32.

Dehner, L.P. and Askin, F.B. (1975) Cytomegalovirus endometritis: report of a case associated with spontaneous abortion. *J. Obstet. Gynecol.*, **45**, 211–14.

Farber, E.R., Leahy, M.S. and Meadows, T.R. (1968) Endometrial blastomycosis acquired by sexual contact. *Obstet. Gynecol.*, **32**, 195–9.

Farooki, M.A. (1967) Epidemiology and pathology of chronic endometritis. *Internat. Surg.*, **48**, 566–73.

Gibbs, R.S., Blanco, J.D., St. Clair, P.J. and Castaneda, Y.S. (1983) *Mycoplasma hominis* and intrauterine infection in late pregnancy. *Sex. Trans. Dis.*, **10**, (suppl. 4), 303–6.

Goldman, R.L. (1970) Herpetic inclusions in the endometrium. *Obstet. Gynecol.*, **36**, 603–5.

Govan, A.D.T. (1962) Tuberculous endometritis. *J. Pathol. Bacteriol.*, **83**, 363–72.

Greenwood, S.M. and Moran, J.J. (1981) Chronic endometritis: morphologic and clinical observations. *Obstet. Gynecol.*, **58**, 176–84.

Gump, D.W., Dickstein, S. and Gibson, M. (1981) Endometritis related to *Chlamydia trachomatis* infection. *Ann. Int. Med.*, **95**, 61–3.

Haines, M. and Stallworthy, J.A. (1952) Genital tuberculosis in the female. *J. Obstet. Gynaecol. Brit. Emp.*, **59**, 721–47.

Hamblen, E.C., Baker, R.D. and Martin, D.S. (1935) Blastomycosis of the female genital tract with report of case. *Am. J. Obstet. Gynecol.*, **30**, 345.

Hart, W.R., Prins, R.P. and Tsai, J.C. (1976) Isolated coccidioidomycosis of the uterus. *Hum. Pathol.*, **7**, 235–9.

Hendrickson, M.R. and Kempson, R.L. (1980) *Surgical Pathology of the Uterine Corpus*, W.B. Saunders, Philadelphia, London, Toronto.

Ho, K-L. (1979) Sarcoidosis of the uterus. *Hum. Pathol.*, **10**, 219–22.

Horne, H.W., Hertig, A.T. and Kundsin, R.B. (1973) Subclinical endometrial inflammation and T-mycoplasma: a possible cause of human reproductive failure. *Int. J. Fertil.*, **18**, 226–31.

Horton, L. and Wilkes, J. (1976) Chronic non-specific endometritis. *Lancet*, **ii**, 366.

Hutchins, C.J. (1977) Tuberculosis of the female genital tract. A changing picture. *Brit. J. Obstet. Gynaecol.*, **84**, 534–8.

Ingerslev, H.J., Møller, B.R. and Mardh, P-A. (1982) *Chlamydia trachomatis* in acute and chronic endometritis. *Scand. J. Infect. Dis.*, **32**, (suppl.), 59–63.

Kitching, A.J. (1984) Endometritis: a clinicopathological and immunohisto-chemical study. BSc. Hons. Thesis, Victoria University of Manchester.

Kurman, R.J. (1982) Benign diseases of the endometrium. In *Pathology of the Female Genital Tract*, 2nd edn, (ed. A. Blaustein), Springer-Verlag, New York, pp. 279–310.

Mardh, P-A, Møller, B.R., Ingerslev, H.J., Nüssler, E., Weström, L. and Wølner-Hanssen, P. (1981) Endometritis caused by *Chlamydia trachomatis*. *Brit. J. Vener. Dis.*, **57**, 191–5.

McCracken, A.W., D'Agostino, A.N., Brucks, A.B. and Kingsley, W.G. (1974) Acquired cytomegalovirus infection presenting as a viral endometritis. *Am. J. Clin. Pathol.*, **61**, 556–60.

Møller, B.R. (1983) The role of mycoplasma in the upper genital tract of women. *Sex Trans. Dis.*, **10** (suppl.4), 281–4.

Molnar, J.J. and Poliak, A. (1983) Recurrent endometrial malakoplakia. *Am. J. Clin. Pathol.*, **80**, 762–4.

Monif, G.R.G. (1981) Recovery of *Neisseria meningitidis* from the cul-de-sac of a woman with endometritis-salpingitis-peritonitis. *Am. J. Obstet. Gynecol.*, **139**, 108–9.

Mouktar, M. (1966) Functional disorders due to bilharzial infection of the female genital tract. *J. Obstet. Gynaecol. Brit. Cwlth.*, **73**, 307–10.

Moyer, D.L. (1975) Endometrial diseases in infertility. In *Progress in Infertility*, 2nd edn (eds S.J. Behrman and R.W. Kistner), Little Brown, Boston, pp. 91–115.

Nogales-Ortiz, F., Taracon, I. and Nogales, F.F. (1979) The pathology of female genital tract tuberculosis. A 31-year study of 1436 cases. *Obstet. Gynecol.*, **53**, 422–8.

Paavonen, J., Miettinen, A., Stevens, C.E., Kiviat, N., Kuo, C-C., Stamm, W.E. and Holmes, K.K. (1983) *Mycoplasma hominis* in cervicitis and endometritis. *Sex. Trans. Dis.*, **10**, (suppl.4), 276–80.

Payan, H., Daino, J. and Kish, M. (1964) Lymphoid follicles in endometrium. *Obstet. Gynecol.*, **23**, 570–73.

Plaut, A. (1950) Human infection with *Cryptococcus glabratus*. Report of case involving uterus and fallopian tube. *Am. J. Clin. Pathol.*, **20**, 377–80.

Rodriguez, M., Okagaki, T. and Richart, R.M. (1972) Mycotic endometritis due to *Candida*, a case report. *Obstet. Gynecol.*, **39**, 292–4.

Rotterdam, H. (1978) Chronic endometritis: a clinicopathologic study. *Pathol. Annual*, **13**, 209–31.

Saw, E.C., Smale, L.E., Einstein, F.H. and Huntington, R.W. (1975) Female genital tract coccidioidomycosis. *Obstet. Gynecol.*, **45**, 199–202.

Schachter, J. (1978) Chlamydial infection. *New Eng. J. Med.*, **298**, 428–35, 490–95, 540–49.

Schaefer, G. (1970) Tuberculosis of the female genital tract. *Clin. Obstet. Gynecol.*, **13**, 965–98.

Schaefer, G., Marcus, R.S. and Kramer, E.E. (1972) Postmenopausal endometrial tuberculosis. *Am. J. Obstet. Gynecol.*, **112**, 681–7.

Schenken, J.R. and Tamisea, J. (1956) *Enterobius vermicularis* (pinworm) infection of the endometrium. *Am. J. Obstet. Gyncecol.*, **72**, 913–14.

Schneider, V., Behm, F.G. and Mumaw, V.T. (1982) Ascending herpetic endometritis. *Obstet. Gynecol.*, **59**, 259–62.

Sen, D.K. and Fox, H. (1967) The lymphoid tissue of the endometrium. *Gynaecologia*, **163**, 371–8.

Thomas, W., Sadeghieh, B., Fresco, R. *et al.* (1978) Malakoplakia of the endometrium, a probable cause of postmenopausal bleeding. *Am. J. Clin. Pathol.*, **69**, 637–41.

Vasudeva, K., Thrasher, T.V. and Richart, R.M. (1972) Chronic endometritis: a clinical and electron microscopic study. *Am. J. Obstet. Gynecol.*, **112**, 749–58.

Weller, T.H. (1971) The cytomegaloviruses: ubiquitous agents with protean clinical manifestations. I. *New Eng. J. Med.*, **285**, 203–14.

Wenkebach, G.F.C. and Curry, B. (1976) Cytomegalovirus infection of the female genital tract. Histologic findings in three cases and review of the literature. *Arch. Pathol. Lab. Med.*, **100**, 609–12.

Weström, L. (1982) Gynecological chlamydial infections. *Infection*, **10** (suppl.), S40–S45.

Williams, A.O. (1967) Pathology of schistosomiasis of the uterine cervix due to *S. haematobium*. *Am. J. Obstet. Gynecol.*, **98**, 784–91.

Winkler, B., Reumann, W., Mitao, M., Gallo, L., Richart, R.M. and Crum, C.P. (1984) Chlamydial endometritis. A histological and immunohistochemical analysis. *Am. J. Surg. Pathol.*, **8**, 771–8.

Wølner-Hanssen, P., Mardh, P-A., Møller, B. and Weström, L. (1982) Endometrial infection in women with *Chlamydial salpingitis*. *Sex. Trans. Dis.*, **9**, 84–8.

8 Miscellaneous benign conditions of the endometrium

The lesions discussed in this chapter have three characteristics in common: they are all benign, all occur in the endometrium and all fall outside the major categories of pathological processes.

8.1 Endometrial changes in uterine prolapse

In most patients with a uterine prolapse the appearances of the endometrium are precisely those which would be expected for the woman's age and hormonal status. In some postmenopausal women, however, the endometrium is less atrophic than would be anticipated and shows an appearance suggestive of persistent low grade oestrogenic stimulation, the glands being lined by a pseudostratified columnar epithelium and sometimes showing weak proliferative activity. These appearances occur in the absence of high oestrogen levels and we have assumed that they are a reactive response to congestion. Whatever their pathogenesis these changes are entirely banal and when encountered in biopsies from patients with a prolapse can safely be ignored, provided of course that a distinction has been drawn between these minor abnormalities and a true endometrial hyperplasia.

8.2 Endometrial abnormalities associated with submucous leiomyomas

The endometrium overlying a small submucous leiomyoma does not differ histologically from that in other areas of the uterine cavity but when the myometrial tumour is large the overlying endometrium may be thinned and represented only by a layer of columnar epithelium with a wisp of subjacent stroma (Figure 1.6). In less extreme cases the overlying endometrium is shallow but contains short, sparse glands or is of moderate thickness and contains glands in which maturation is delayed relative to the endometrium elsewhere in the uterine cavity. Hence, in biopsy specimens the admixture of endometrium overlying a large

130

submucous leiomyoma with endometrium from elsewhere in the uterine cavity may produce a confusing picture which can lead to an erroneous diagnosis of luteal inadequacy. Not uncommonly, however, fragments of the underlying leiomyoma are included in such biopsy specimens and these may yield a clue to the true diagnosis.

8.3 Endometrial metaplasia

Metaplastic changes occur with some frequency in the endometrium (Table 8.1), particularly in its epithelial component (Hendrickson and Kempson, 1980); these are of no clinical importance but may give rise to diagnostic confusion when encountered in biopsies.

The high incidence of metaplasia in the endometrium is, to a considerable extent, an eloquent tribute to the plasticity of Müllerian ductal derivatives, undifferentiated cells in such tissues having a potentiality to differentiate along any of the various Müllerian pathways. Thus undifferentiated stem cells in endometrial epithelium can differentiate along endometrial lines but can also pursue alternative tubal or endocervical pathways with resulting tubal (ciliated cell) or mucinous metaplasia. Müllerian tissues also have a marked capacity for squamous metaplasia and can undergo intestinal metaplasia.

Some alterations in endometrial cell morphology, such as eosinophilic or surface syncytial-like change, have sometimes been included within the general concept of endometrial metaplasias but appear to us to fall outside the definition of a metaplastic change; these are therefore considered separately in a later portion of this chapter.

Metaplastic changes may be encountered in normally cycling, atrophic, hyperplastic or neoplastic endometria and their presence, though sometimes confusing, does not alter or modify the primary histological diagnosis of the state of the endometrium.

Table 8.1 Classification of endometrial metaplasias

Epithelial metaplasias
Squamous metaplasia and morule formation
Ciliated cell metaplasia
Mucinous metaplasia
Hob nail metaplasia
Clear cell metaplasia
Gastrointestinal metaplasia

Stromal metaplasias
Myomatous metaplasia
Osseous metaplasia
Chrondroid metaplasia

8.3.1   Epithelial metaplasias

(*a*)   *Squamous metaplasia and morule formation*   Squamous metaplasia is extremely common in the endometrium (Baggish and Woodruff, 1967) and areas of such metaplasia may show overt evidence of squamous differentiation (Figure 8.1), such as keratinization or intercellular bridge formation, or can take the form of morules (Dutra, 1959). These latter (Figure 8.2) are rounded or ovoid aggregates of cells which have indistinct margins, a modest amount of eosinophilic cytoplasm and rounded, ovoid or spindly nuclei. Central necrosis is sometimes seen in large morules but the cells in a morule are always cytologically bland and usually devoid of mitotic activity. Morules can show focal squamous differentiation and it is generally believed that they represent a form of immature squamous metaplasia.

Both squamous metaplasia and morules usually occur within the endometrial glands, the metaplastic cells blending with the glandular epithelial cells and tending to fill, partially or completely, the glandular lumens. Foci of both squamous metaplasia and morules, particularly the latter, can, however, expand to an extent that they obliterate both the lumens and the lining epithelium of the glands in which they have arisen,

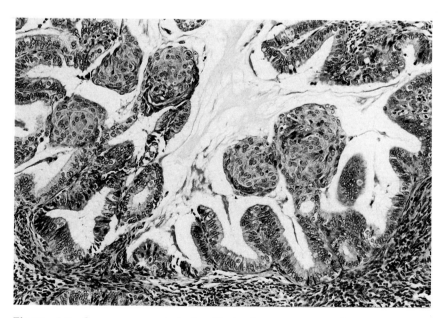

Figure 8.1 Squamous metaplasia. Foci of mature metaplastic squamous epithelium are present in the columnar epithelium of this hyperplastic endometrium. Haematoxylin and Eosin × 186.

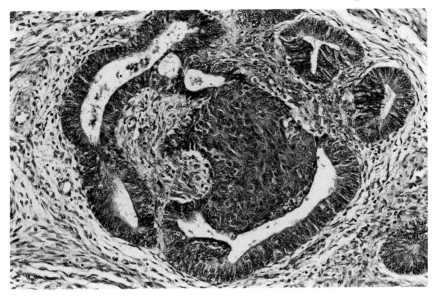

Figure 8.2 Squamous metaplasia. A gland in an endometrial polyp, exhibiting mild complex hyperplasia, contains a squamous morule. Haematoxylin and Eosin × 186.

subsequent fusion of squamous or morular masses then resulting in the formation of sheets of metaplastic cells. Rather uncommonly, metaplastic squamous tissue is seen on the outer aspect of the glandular epithelium, forming a focus which bulges into the stroma.

Although squamous metaplasia occurs most frequently within the endometrial glands it is also seen in, and is sometimes confined to, the surface epithelium; occasionally the entire surface epithelium is replaced by metaplastic squamous epithelium (Figure 8.3), this condition of 'ichthyosis uteri' being seen most commonly in, but by no means being confined to, elderly women with pyometra.

Intraglandular squamous metaplasia, cytologically bland and devoid of mitotic activity, usually presents few diagnostic difficulties in biopsies. If such metaplasia occurs, however, in adenocarcinomatous acini it is important to distinguish between the bland tissue and the malignant squamous epithelium which forms one component of an adenosquamous carcinoma, a distinction discussed in Chapter 10.

Morules pose a wider range of diagnostic possibilities. When growing in sheets, and especially if showing central necrosis, they may resemble poorly differentiated solid adenocarcinoma but consideration of the bland nature of the morular cells and their lack of mitotic activity should

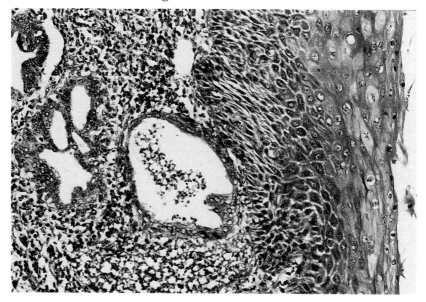

Figure 8.3   Squamous metaplasia. The surface epithelium of the endometrium, to the right, is replaced by a mature, stratified squamous epithelium. The underlying endometrium is inactive and the stroma infiltrated by chronic inflammatory cells. Haematoxylin and Eosin × 186.

lead to avoidance of a diagnostic error. Morules can, perhaps somewhat surprisingly, bear a resemblance to epithelioid granulomas but the type of cell involved and the absence of any rim of surrounding chronic inflammatory cells should make the distinction between these two conditions a relatively easy task. Morules with spindly nuclei can mimic a focus of smooth muscle metaplasia or a stromal nodule from which they differ, however, in their lack of individual cell reticulin envelopment, their positive staining for keratins and their negative reaction for vimentin.

Curettings from cases of ichthyosis uteri may yield endometrium together with isolated strips of mature squamous epithelium. It is natural in such circumstances to conclude, despite any protestations from the gynaecologist, that the squamous tissue is derived from the cervix rather than from the uterine cavity and in most biopsies showing this pattern that conclusion will indeed be correct. The possibility of an ichthyosis uteri, should, however, always be borne in mind, particularly in elderly women, and mentioned in the report. If curettings contain benign squamous epithelium which clearly overlies subjacent endometrial glands the diagnosis of ichthyosis uteri will present no difficulties.

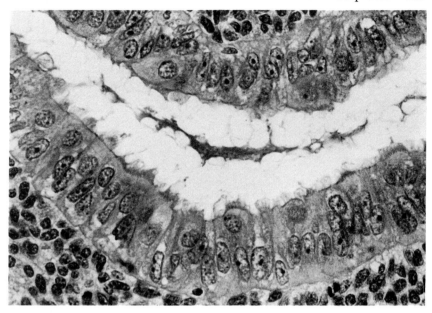

Figure 8.4 Ciliated cell metaplasia in an endometrium showing simple hyperplasia. The gland is lined by an almost pure population of ciliated cells. Note that despite the mild pseudostratification of the epithelium there is no evidence of cytological atypia: perinuclear cytoplasmic clearing is quite prominent. Haematoxylin and Eosin × 465.

(*b*)   *Ciliated cell (tubal) metaplasia*   Strictly speaking the term 'metaplasia' should not be used to describe the presence of ciliated cells in endometrial glandular epithelium for such cells are a normal constitutent of this epithelium, particularly during the proliferative phase of the menstrual cycle (Fruin and Tighe, 1967). Ciliated cell metaplasia describes, however, the situation, encountered most commonly in endometria subjected to prolonged unopposed oestrogenic stimulation, in which pyramidal ciliated cells predominate in the epithelial lining of an endometrial gland (Figure 8.4) or group of glands (Hendrickson and Kempson, 1980). These ciliated cells have eosinophilic, often vacuolated, cytoplasm and central round or ovoid nuclei. A perinuclear clearing of the cytoplasm ('perinuclear halo') is quite commonly seen. There is a tendency for these ciliated cells to stratify and they may form intraglandular tufts or papillae. Any confusion with a neoplastic process should be dispelled by the bland nature of the cells and their lack of mitotic figures.

(*c*)   *Mucinous metaplasia*   The lining of a single endometrial gland, of a group of endometrial glands or, occasionally, of the entire endometrial

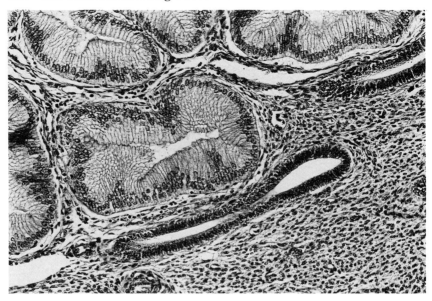

Figure 8.5 Mucinous metaplasia. The glands, in the lower part of the field, are lined by cubo-columnar cells with scanty cytoplasm which show neither secretory nor proliferative activity. The glands in the upper part of the field are lined by tall, mucus-secreting columnar cells of the type found in the endocervix. There is no cytological atypia. Haematoxylin and Eosin × 186.

glandular population may be replaced by an epithelium which is histologically identical to that of the endocervix (Hendrickson and Kempson, 1980; Desmopoulos and Greco, 1983). Such an epithelium is formed by columnar cells with central or basal, regular nuclei and abundant clear cytoplasm which stains positively for mucin (Figure 8.5). The mucinous epithelium is usually non-stratified but can show pseudostratification, budding and papillary projections. Occasionally, the surface, rather than the glandular epithelium undergoes mucinous metaplasia (Figure 8.6).

Mucinous metaplasia occurs predominantly in postmenopausal women and can, when extensive, be associated with a mucometra. When seen in curettings mucinous metaplasia has to be distinguished from endocervical glandular epithelium. This is only possible if a direct transition from endometrial to mucinous epithelium can be traced, if the surrounding stroma is of endometrial rather than endocervical type or if there is an admixture within a single tissue fragment, in a specimen which is not from the isthmic area, of glands lined by endometrial-type and mucinous-type epithelium.

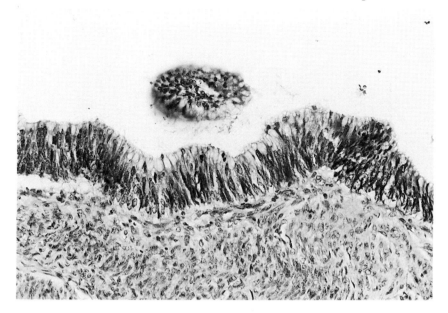

Figure 8.6 Mucinous metaplasia. In this hysterectomy specimen the uterine body was lined by a stratified mucinous epithelium which replaced the endometrium. Haematoxylin and Eosin × 232.

(*d*) *Hob nail metaplasia*   This very rare endometrial metaplastic change is characterized by the presence of cells having a typical 'hob nail' appearance which replace, to a variable degree, the normal, glandular epithelium (Fechner, 1968). These cells have a 'teardrop' appearance with their narrow point towards the basal lamina; the cells are cytologically bland with dense regular nuclei and clear or eosinophilic cytoplasm. The lack of any cytological atypia and of mitotic activity serves to distinguish these metaplastic cells from those seen in a clear cell adenocarcinoma of the endometrium.

(*e*) *Clear cell metaplasia*   In this extremely uncommon form of endometrial metaplasia cuboidal cells with strikingly clear cytoplasm focally replace endometrial glandular epithelium (Hendrickson and Kempson, 1980). These cells contain glycogen and small amounts of mucin. The lack of any cytological atypia allows for a distinction from a clear cell adenocarcinoma whilst the absence of decidual change and of hypersecretory epithelium, typical of pregnancy, excludes a diagnosis of Arias-Stella change.

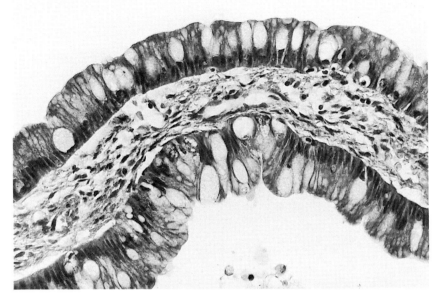

Figure 8.7 Enteric metaplasia. The epithelium in this endometrium was replaced focally by an enteric epithelium containing goblet cells. Mucin stains showed a specific intestinal pattern. Haematoxylin and Eosin × 370.

(*f*) *Intestinal metaplasia* Very occasionally intestinal metaplasia is encountered in the endometrium (Figure 8.7). The metaplastic epithelium is formed principally of columnar cells with ovoid nuclei and a prominent brush border. Interspersed with these are enteric-type goblet cells whilst argyrophil cells may also be present. The goblet cells give a strongly positive reaction with the periodate borohydrate/potassium hydroxide/PAS stain, thus indicating that they contain *o*-acetylated sialomucins of enteric type (Tiltman and Wells, in prep.).

8.3.2   Stromal metaplasias

(*a*) *Cartilaginous metaplasia* Foci of mature cartilage are occasionally found in the endometrial stroma (Roth and Taylor, 1966). It is often possible to trace a peripheral transition between the surrounding stromal cells and the metaplastic cartilaginous cells.

Metaplastic cartilage must be differentiated from fetal remnants; the observation of a transition from stromal to cartilaginous cells at the margin of the focus, the absence of any other tissue elements and the lack of a recent history of pregnancy or abortion would all favour a diagnosis of metaplasia rather than fetal implantation. Metaplastic cartilage has also to be distinguished from that found as a heterologous element in some mixed Müllerian tumours. The absence of any other tissues and of any evidence of a neoplastic process makes this distinction an easy one.

(b) *Osseous metaplasia (Figure 8.8)*   Metaplastic bone formation is sometimes seen in the endometrial stroma (Ganem *et al.*, 1962; Courpas *et al.*, 1964; Shatia and Hoshika, 1982) and, as with cartilaginous metaplasia, there is often a traceable transition between endometrial stromal cells and osseous cells at the periphery of the bony focus. Osseous metaplasia tends to occur in a setting of acute or chronic endometritis and is particularly associated with post-abortal infections.

The differential diagnosis of osseous metaplasia is, as with cartilaginous metaplasia, from fetal remnants and from bone which is present as a heterologous element in a mixed Müllerian tumour. The criteria for distinguishing these conditions are the same as those outlined above for cartilaginous metaplasia.

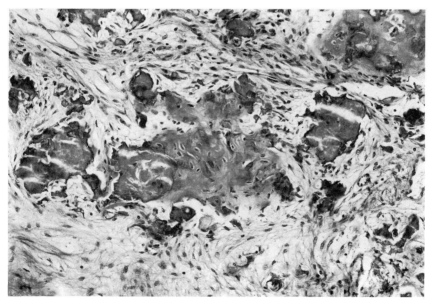

Figure 8.8   Osseous metaplasia. Patchy calcification and focal osteoid metaplasia in the stroma of an endometrium which is extensively fibrosed. Haematoxylin and Eosin × 186.

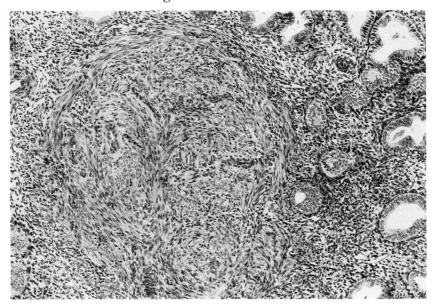

Figure 8.9 Smooth muscle metaplasia. A discrete focus of leiomyomatous metaplasia is present in the endometrium and is compressing the surrounding glands and stroma. The focus was identified in a patient with menorrhagia. Haematoxylin and Eosin × 117.

(c) *Smooth muscle metaplasia* The endometrial stroma can contain small nodules of smooth muscle which compress the surrounding tissue and are not connected with the underlying superficial myometrium (Figure 8.9). These have been classed as 'intraendometrial leiomyomas' but are more probably a result of stromal smooth muscle metaplasia (Bird and Willis, 1965).

Nodular smooth muscle metaplasia in the endometrium has to be distinguished from a stromal nodule and this can only be achieved by recognizing that the constituent cells are of smooth muscle, rather than stromal, type. The distinction between smooth muscle and stromal tumours, in both morphological and immunocytochemical terms, is discussed in Chapter 11 and it must be emphasized that this differentiation is critically important in biopsies. Both stromal nodules and nodular smooth muscle metaplasia are benign conditions but the presence of a stromal lesion, no matter how apparently banal, necessitates hysterectomy to exclude a low grade endometrial stromal sarcoma whilst smooth muscle metaplasia merits no treatment.

8.4   Cytological abnormalities

8.4.1   *Surface syncytial-like change*

The cells of the endometrial surface epithelium may, on occasion, show papillary proliferation (Hendrickson and Kempson, 1980). The papillae consist of cytologically bland cells with ovoid, rounded or pyknotic nuclei, indistinct margins and a moderate amount of eosinophilic cytoplasm (Figure 8.10). The papillae are devoid of any stromal support and the lack of definition of the cell margins imparts to them a syncytial-like appearance. This papillary syncytial-like change may extend into the superficial portion of adjacent glands and, characteristically, the papillary aggregates are focally or diffusely infiltrated by polymorphonuclear leucocytes. It is probable that this change represents, in fact, a very early stage of surface squamous metaplasia.

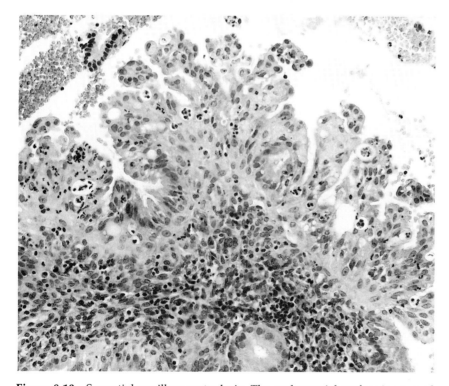

Figure 8.10   Syncytial papillary metaplasia. The endometrial surface is covered by epithelial cells that form a syncytial-like mass with indistinct cell borders. The nuclei are bland. The underlying stroma is chronically inflamed. Haematoxylin and Eosin × 230 approx. Photograph kindly supplied by Dr R.L. Kempson.

Surface syncytial-like change can, when encountered in curettings, bear some resemblance to a papillary adenocarcinoma of the endometrium. Disastrous over-diagnosis of this clinically unimportant abnormality can be averted by taking note of the bland nature of the cells in surface syncytial-like change.

8.4.2   *Eosinophilic change*

Epithelial cells in an endometrium occasionally have small, round, basophilic nuclei and markedly eosinophilic cytoplasm. Whether these cells are oncocytes has not yet been determined but their presence has no clinical significance.

8.5   Fetal remnants

Following abortion, either spontaneous or induced, fetal tissue can remain embedded in the endometrium (Newton and Abell, 1972; Tyagi *et al.*, 1979). Bleeding, after a period of months or even years, may

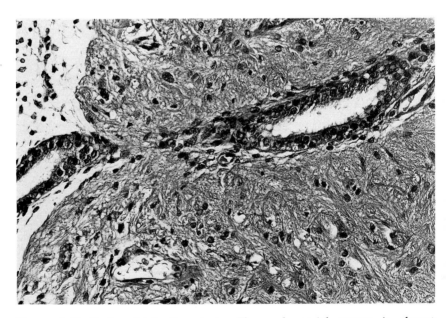

Figure 8.11 Endometrial gliomatosis. The endometrial stroma is almost completely replaced by glial tissue. The distinctly fibrillar structure of the tissue is apparent and the endometrial gland which traverses the field is of normal appearance. Haematoxylin and Eosin × 297.

complicate the implantation of such fetal tissues and curettage under these circumstances will yield endometrium admixed with a melange of fetal tissues such as cartilage, bone, glial tissue, kidney, liver, skin and retina.

Clearly, these findings may give rise to a suspicion of a uterine teratoma and, indeed, it is almost certain that many of the reported cases of teratomatous neoplasms of the uterus were in fact examples of fetal remnants. A distinction of fetal remnants from a teratoma rests upon the usually intimate admixture of the fetal tissues with endometrium and upon the pattern of the implanted tissues which usually differs markedly from that seen in a teratoma.

In some cases fetal remnants within the endometrium are represented only by glial tissue (Zettergren, 1973; Niven and Stansfeld, 1973; Roca et al., 1980), a condition sometimes known as endometrial gliomatosis (Figure 8.11). The glial tissue usually forms well-defined islands, may become polypoid and occasionally bears a slight resemblance to decidua. Staining for glial fibrillary acidic protein will resolve any doubts as to the nature of the tissue.

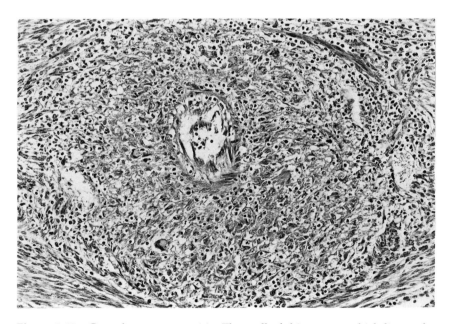

Figure 8.12 Granulomatous arteritis. The wall of this artery, which lies at the junction of the basalis and myometrium, is diffusely infiltrated by non-caseating granulomatous tissue in which macrophage giant cells are seen. The arterial wall is disrupted. Haematoxylin and Eosin × 186.

8.6   Vasculitis

Giant cell arteritis can affect the vasculature of the uterus (Pirozynski, 1976; Petrides *et al.*, 1979). The vascular lesions may be limited to the arteries within the myometrium (Figure 8.12) but can extend to involve the spiral arteries in the endometrium and thus be apparent in curettage specimens. Involved endometrial arteries show replacement of their walls by granulomatous tissue and the appearances may at first sight resemble those of a tuberculous granuloma. Elastic stains will, however, demonstrate the presence of a vessel in the centre of the inflammatory focus, even when the disease is well advanced with marked vascular destruction. In patients with a giant cell arteritis a systemic disease, such as temporal arteritis or polymyalgia rheumatica, should be suspected. A necrotizing arteritis of the medium and small muscular arteries of the uterus can occur as a localized lesion and is sometimes encountered in women suffering from polyarteritis nodosa.

8.7   Endometrial polyps

The term 'polyp' is purely descriptive and does not, in itself, denote any specific histological process; thus an endometrial neoplasm or a submucous leiomyoma may well present as a polypoid mass within the uterus. By convention, however, the term 'endometrial polyp' is generally taken as referring to a focal, circumscribed overgrowth of the mucosa, usually the basal portion, which protrudes into the uterine cavity. It is thought that such polyps form either because of a focal hypersensitivity to oestrogen or a local insensitivity to progesterone. Polyps do not occur before the menarche but increase in frequency thereafter to reach a peak incidence during the fifth decade.

8.7.1   Simple polyps

As seen in curettings, simple endometrial polyps are formed of endometrial glands set in a stroma that is at least partially fibrous (Figure 8.13). Those originating from the isthmic area may contain an admixture of endometrial and endocervical glands. The endometrial glands in a polyp do not usually share in the normal cyclical activity of the endometrium and are often either inactive or only weakly proliferative. Simple hyperplasia, focal complex hyperplasia or focal atypical hyperplasia, limited to the glands in the polyp, are sometimes seen. In postmenopausal women the glands are inactive and can show senile cystic change, this latter phenomenon probably reflecting more the tendency of foci of senile cystic change to become polypoid rather than the development of cystic change in the glands of a pre-existing polyp.

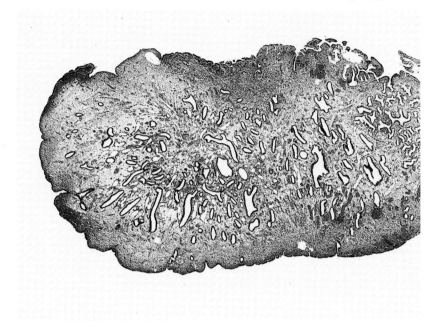

Figure 8.13   Endometrial polyp. A typical, benign polyp composed of functional and basal endometrium. There is a mild degree of glandular architectural atypia. Haematoxylin and Eosin × 18.5.

Glandular secretory activity is seen in a small proportion of polyps but is usually patchy, weak and irregular.

The stroma of a simple polyp, as already remarked, invariably contains at least some fibrous tissue and this, together with the characteristic presence of a leash or cluster of small, thick-walled vessels (Figure 8.14), usually in the base or stalk but sometimes seen in the body of the polyp, is of considerable diagnostic value in recognizing a polyp in curettings. Reliance for making this diagnosis should not be placed on the presence of surface epithelium on three or all sides of a tissue fragment for a similar appearance can be seen in polypoidal pieces of normal endometrium.

A simple polyp may undergo haemorrhage, infarction or apical ulceration but there is usually a sufficient retention of the histological pattern to allow for diagnosis. The cardinal characteristics of stromal fibrous tissue and the presence of thick-walled vessels distinguish a simple polyp from a polypoidal piece of normal endometrium whilst the Müllerian adenofibroma, with which a simple polyp can be confused, usually has club-shaped papillary projections into cystic spaces (Figure 11.8).

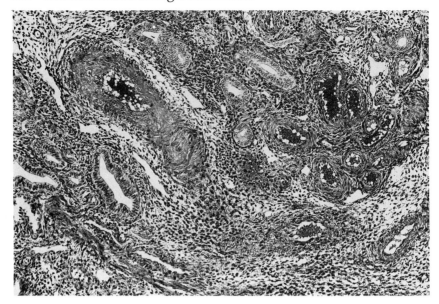

Figure 8.14   Endometrial polyp. A cluster of thick-walled arteries is seen in the core of the polyp. Haematoxylin and Eosin × 93.

Adenocarcinomatous change in a polyp is very uncommon, many reported examples of the phenomenon being, in reality, adenocarcinomas growing in a polypoidal fashion (Salm, 1972). To establish that an adenocarcinoma has arisen in a pre-existing polyp it is necessary to demonstrate that the malignant tissue is separated from normal endometrium by the base and stalk of the polyp, these latter showing no malignant features. It is commonly not possible to make a topographic analysis of this nature in curettage material.

8.7.2   Adenofibromatous polyps

These differ from simple polyps only in the fact that their stroma consists solely of fibrous tissue.

8.7.3   Adenomyomatous polyps

These uncommon polyps contain bands of smooth muscle in their stroma. It is not clear whether these muscular elements represent superficial myometrium which was originally admixed with the basal endometrium or smooth muscle metaplasia in the stroma of a simple polyp.

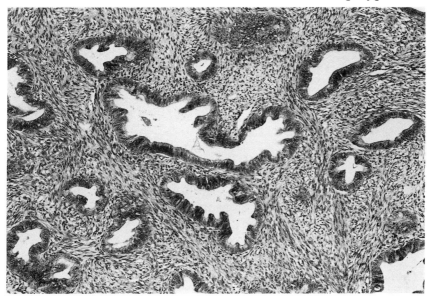

Figure 8.15 Atypical adenomyomatous polyp. The glands are irregular in contour exhibiting in-foldings, epithelial budding and out-pouchings. The stroma is formed predominantly of smooth muscle. Haematoxylin and Eosin × 93.

(a) *Atypical polypoid adenomyoma* (Figure 8.15). This term has been applied to adenomyomatous polyps in which the glandular component shows a variable degree of architectural and cytological atypia (Mazur, 1981; Young *et al.*, 1986). These polyps can, in curettings, be mistaken for adenocarcinomas which are infiltrating myometrium. The stromal smooth muscle of the atypical polypoid adenomyoma rarely has, however, the fasciculated pattern of true myometrium, the fibres tending to be arranged in a haphazard fashion. Furthermore the smooth muscle fibres are commonly admixed with fibrous tissue and there may also be a minor endometrial stromal component.

Despite their slightly alarming appearance atypical polypoid adenomyomas appear to behave in a benign fashion, though they may well regrow if incompletely removed.

8.7.4 Stromatous polyps

These are exceptionally rare and consist only of endometrial stroma. It is virtually impossible in curettage material to distinguish polyps of this type from an endometrial stromal sarcoma.

148 Miscellaneous benign conditions

References

Baggish, M.S. and Woodruff, J.D. (1967) The occurrence of squamous epithelium in the endometrium. *Obstet. Gynecol. Surv.*, **22**, 69–115.

Bird, C.C. and Willis, R.A. (1965) The production of smooth muscle by the endometrial stroma of the adult human uterus. *J. Pathol. Bacteriol.*, **90**, 75–81.

Courpas, A.S., Morris, J.D. and Woodruff, J.D. (1964) Osteoid tissue in utero: report of three cases. *Obstet. Gynecol.*, **24**, 636–40.

Desmopoulos, R.I. and Greco, M.A. (1983) Mucinous metaplasia of the endometrium: ultrastructural and histochemical characteristics. *Int. J. Gynecol. Pathol.*, **1**, 383–90.

Dutra, F. (1959) Intraglandular morules of the endometrium. *Am. J. Clin. Pathol.*, **31**, 60–65.

Fechner, R.E. (1968) Endometrium with pattern of mesonephroma (report of a case). *Obstet. Gynecol.*, **31**, 485–90.

Fruin, A.H. and Tighe, J.R. (1967) Tubal metaplasia of the endometrium. *J. Obstet. Gynaecol. Brit. Cwlth.*, **74**, 93–7.

Ganem, K.J., Parsons, L. and Friedell, G. (1962) Endometrial ossification. *Am. J. Obstet. Gynecol.*, **83**, 1592–4.

Hendrickson, M.R. and Kempson, R.L. (1980) Endometrial epithelial metaplasias: report of 89 cases and proposed classification. *Am. J. Surg. Pathol.*, **4**, 525–42.

Mazur, M.T. (1981) Atypical polypoid adenomyomas of the endometrium. *Am. J. Surg. Pathol.*, **5**, 473–82.

Newton, C.W. and Abell, M.R. (1972) Iatrogenic fetal implants. *Obstet. Gynecol.*, **40**, 686–91.

Niven, P.A.R. and Stansfeld, A.G. (1973) 'Glioma' of the uterus: a fetal homograft. *Am. J. Obstet. Gynecol.*, **115**, 534–8.

Petrides, M., Robertson, I.G. and Fox, H. (1979) Giant cell arteritis of the female genital tract. *Br. J. Obstet. Gynecol.*, **86**, 148–51.

Pirozynski, W.J. (1976) Giant cell arteritis of the uterus: report of two cases. *Am. J. Clin. Pathol.*, **65**, 308–13.

Roca, A.N., Guarjardo, M. and Estrada, W.J. (1980) Glial polyp of the cervix and endometrium. *Am. J. Clin. Pathol.*, **73**, 718–20.

Roth, E. and Taylor, H.B. (1966) Heterotopic cartilage in uterus. *Obstet. Gynecol.*, **27**, 838–44.

Salm, R. (1972) The incidence and significance of early carcinomas in endometrial polyps. *J. Pathol.*, **108**, 47–54.

Shatia, N.N. and Hoshika, M.G. (1982) Uterine osseous metaplasia. *Obstet. Gynecol.*, **60**, 256–9.

Tyagi, S.P., Saxena, K., Rizvi, R. and Langley, F.A. (1979) Foetal remnants in the uterus and their relation to other uterine heterotopias. *Histopathology*, **3**, 339–45.

Young, R.H., Treger, T. and Scully, R.E. (1986) Atypical polypoid adenomyomas of the uterus: a report of 27 cases. *Am. J. Clin. Pathol.*, **86**, 139–45.

Zettergren, L. (1973) Glial tissue in the uterus. *Am. J. Pathol.*, **71**, 419–26.

9 Endometrial hyperplasias and intra-endometrial adenocarcinoma

9.1 Classification of endometrial hyperplasias

A pathologist confronted with the task of recognizing and categorizing the various forms of endometrial hyperplasia, as seen in curettage material, must work within the framework of a classification of these conditions. Unfortunately, no generally agreed classification of hyperplastic abnormalities of the endometrium exists and, indeed, the entire topic has become confused almost to the point of anarchy by a plethora of proposed classifications and by a complicated and inconsistent nomenclature.

In reality, the only important distinction, in both prognostic and therapeutic terms, between the various forms of endometrial hyperplasia is between those which are associated with a significant risk of evolving into an endometrial adenocarcinoma and those devoid of any such risk. There is now quite widespread agreement that the defining and only feature of an endometrial hyperplasia which is indicative of a potentiality for malignant change is cytological atypia (Welch and Scully, 1977; Fox and Buckley, 1982; Kurman *et al.*, 1985; Norris *et al.*, 1986) and hence the fundamental subdivision of the endometrial hyperplasias is into those with cytological atypia and those lacking this feature. From a prognostic viewpoint this is a fully adequate classification but one which is possibly too stark for diagnostic purposes in so far as hyperplasias without cytological atypia may involve both glands and stroma or may be confined solely to the glands.

The recommended classification of the endometrial hyperplasias is therefore that shown in Table 9.1 in which hyperplasia with cytological atypia is classed as 'atypical hyperplasia' and hyperplasias lacking cytological atypia are subdivided into 'simple' and 'complex' forms (Norris *et al.*, 1986). Whilst not being fully in sympathy with the conceptual approach on which this classification is based we do, nevertheless, accept that it is prognostically valid and easy to apply in practice. The terminology used in this classification, though not without

149

Table 9.1 Classification of
endometrial hyperplasias

Simple hyperplasia
Complex hyperplasia
Atypical hyperplasia

its critics, is straightforward and uncomplicated. The condition of 'simple hyperplasia' corresponds to that often classed as 'cystic glandular hyperplasia'. The latter is an inappropriate form of nomenclature since this type of hyperplasia is not restricted to the glandular component of the endometrium; further, the glands are not necessarily cystic in appearance. A simple hyperplasia is sometimes called 'a disordered proliferative endometrium' (Hendrickson and Kempson, 1987) but we feel that this term, if used at all, should be restricted to the earliest, and mildest, stages of a simple hyperplasia.

A complex hyperplasia corresponds to glandular hyperplasia with architectural atypia. Some authors define a complex hyperplasia in terms of both glandular crowding and architectural atypia (Norris *et al.*, 1986) but, whilst agreeing that glandular crowding is usually present, we accept architectural atypia as the defining feature of this form of endometrial hyperplasia.

We have elaborated elsewhere (Fox and Buckley, 1982) our reasons for believing that the endometrial abnormality usually classed as a hyperplasia with cytological atypia is in fact a form of intraendometrial neoplasia rather than a true hyperplasia. We persist in this belief but long-held attitudes in pathology are difficult to alter and the concept of intraendometrial neoplasia has not gained widespread acceptance, despite the overwhelming scientific evidence for its validity. We accept therefore, albeit with considerable reluctance, the use of the term 'atypical hyperplasia' to describe those proliferative endometrial lesions which, whilst showing cellular atypia, fall short of being genuine adenocarcinomas.

The term 'adenomatous hyperplasia' should have no place in any contemporary classification of endometrial hyperplasias. This diagnostic label has been used so indiscriminately as to have lost any meaning it may once have had and is, furthermore, indefensible in both conceptual and semantic terms.

Secretory change may be superimposed on any form of hyperplasia if, for instance, a progestagen is given or if ovulation occurs after a series of anovulatory cycles. We do not recognize, however, any specific condition of 'secretory hyperplasia'.

9.2   Histological appearances of the various forms of endometrial hyperplasia

9.2.1   *Simple hyperplasia*

This condition represents the physiological response of the endometrium to prolonged, unopposed oestrogenic stimulation, whether this be of endogenous (repeated anovulatory cycles, oestrogenic ovarian tumour, polycystic ovary syndrome) or exogenous (administration of oestrogens without a progestagen) origin. It is a true hyperplasia with an increase in endometrial bulk and hence curettings from women with this condition tend to be bulky and sometimes polypoid. The tissue often has a somewhat velvety appearance and tiny cystic spaces may be apparent even on naked-eye examination. Simple hyperplasia is a diffuse process which involves the entire endometrium with resulting loss of the distinction between basal and functional zones. This will not, of course, be apparent in curettage material but nevertheless the biopsied tissue will show throughout the appearance of a simple hyperplasia, there being no admixture of hyperplastic and non-hyperplastic endometrium and no

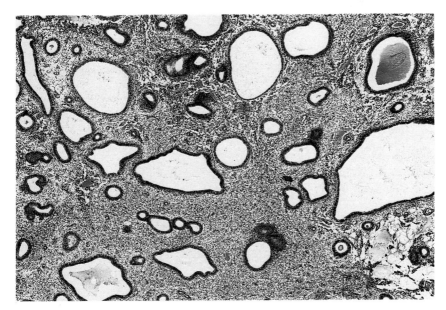

Figure 9.1 Simple hyperplasia. This is characterized by great variability in glandular size. Some glands are large and cystically dilated whilst others are of normal or even unusually small size. The stroma is cellular. The normal gland to stroma ratio is maintained. Haematoxylin and Eosin × 37.

basal type endometrium. The endometrial glands show a proliferative pattern but vary markedly in calibre (Figure 9.1), some being unusually large, others of approximately normal diameter and yet others unduly small; it is this variability in size, rather than just the presence of glands which appear dilated, which is the characteristic feature of this form of endometrial hyperplasia. The glands often have a smooth rounded contour though some degree of budding into the stroma is not uncommon. The glandular epithelium (Figure 9.2) is formed by plump, regular tall cuboidal or low columnar cells which have strongly basophilic cytoplasm and round, basally or centrally sited nuclei. There is commonly a minor or moderate degree of multilayering but intraluminal tufting, loss of polarity and cytological atypia are not seen. The glands may show quite well marked tubal or squamous metaplasia, the latter often taking the form of morules. Eosinophilic cell change is not uncommon.

In a simple hyperplasia the stroma shares in the hyperplastic process and hence the gland-to-stroma ratio is normal, there being no glandular

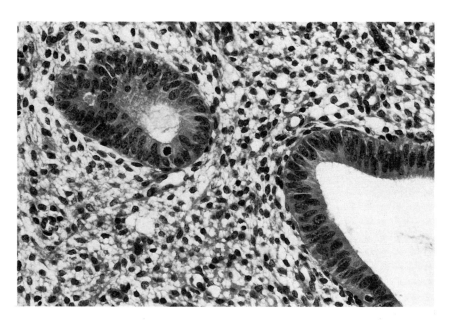

Figure 9.2   Simple hyperplasia. The stroma is cellular and of the type seen in the normal follicular phase. The glands are lined by an epithelium which is pseudostratified, contains occasional mitoses, resembles that seen in the proliferative phase and shows no evidence of cytological atypia. Haematoxylin and Eosin × 370.

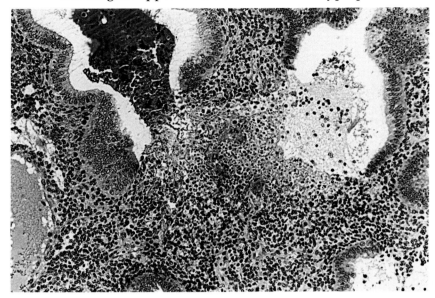

Figure 9.3 Simple hyperplasia. An area of necrosis which is infiltrated by polymorphonuclear leucocytes. Haematoxylin and Eosin × 186.

crowding. The stroma usually appears hypercellular and often shows the 'naked nuclei' appearance characteristic of a proliferative phase endometrium. Focal areas of necrosis may be present in the stroma (Figure 9.3) and these are often infiltrated by inflammatory cells; small collections of foamy stromal histiocytes are not uncommonly seen. Dilated sub-epithelial sinusoidal vascular spaces are a characteristic feature of a simple hyperplasia but these will rarely be apparent in biopsy specimens.

Mitotic figures, both in the glands and in the stroma, may be abundant or sparse but are invariably of normal form.

Episodic bleeding, often severe and prolonged, occurs in women with a simple endometrial hyperplasia. It is assumed, perhaps rather simplistically, that this is due either to an intermittent waning of oestrogen levels or to the endometrium reaching a bulk that surpasses the supportive capacity of the oestrogens. Curettage in such cases may reveal a surprisingly undisturbed picture of simple hyperplasia or may show a necrotic, haemorrhagic endometrium with a shrunken stroma and collapsed glands. The circumference of the latter may suggest, however, that some of these had been cystically dilated.

9.2.2 *Complex hyperplasia*

This endometrial abnormality may occur under the same conditions as does a simple hyperplasia, i.e. in the endometrium exposed to unopposed oestrogenic stimulation, but can also develop in normally cycling or atrophic endometria. A complex hyperplasia is restricted to the glandular component of the endometrium and does not involve the stroma. Furthermore, the hyperplastic process is almost invariably focal rather than generalized, hence curettings from cases of complex hyperplasia are not usually unduly bulky and commonly contain an admixture of hyperplastic and normal endometrium. The hyperplastic glands are variable in size but are often larger and more numerous than normal with consequent crowding and a reduction in the amount of intervening stroma. By definition, there is an abnormal pattern of glandular growth with outpouchings, or budding, of the glandular epithelium into the surrounding stroma (Figure 9.4) to produce the 'finger-in-glove' pattern. In biopsies, the glands may be cut longitudinally and multiple outpouchings can impart a serrated pattern which may be confused with that of a normal late secretory endometrium (Figure 9.5). Papillary projections of cells, with connective tissue cores,

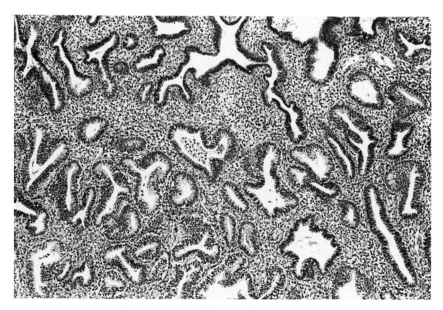

Figure 9.4 Complex hyperplasia. The glands are rather crowded, irregular in contour and exhibit budding and out pouchings. Haematoxylin and Eosin × 93.

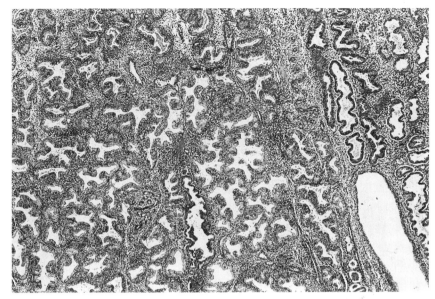

Figure 9.5 Complex hyperplasia. The endometrial glands to the left of the field are closely packed and resemble those of the late secretory phase, having irregular contours, infolding of the epithelium and out pouchings. Haematoxylin and Eosin × 37.

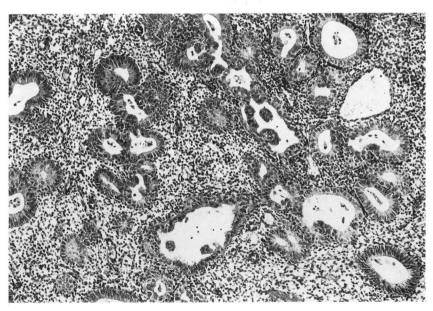

Figure 9.6 Complex hyperplasia. The glands to the right exhibit prominent budding of their epithelium and there is some loss of nuclear polarity. Haematoxylin and Eosin × 117.

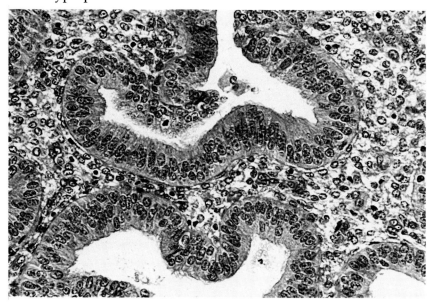

Figure 9.7 Complex hyperplasia. The cells lining the glands are similar in appearance to those seen in simple hyperplasia (Figure 9.2). There is no evidence of cytological atypia. Haematoxylin and Eosin × 370.

into the glandular lumena are not uncommon and tangential cutting of these may give an impression of solid buds of cells extending into the glands (Figure 9.6). The glandular epithelium is regular (Figure 9.7) and formed of tall cuboidal or low columnar cells with ovoid or, less commonly, rounded basal or central nuclei. Nucleoli are inconspicuous, cellular atypia is absent, multilayering is minimal and there is no loss of nuclear polarity. The stroma between the hyperplastic glands is commonly compressed but is not hypercellular. Mitotic figures may be fairly numerous in the glandular epithelium and are of normal form.

9.2.3   Atypical hyperplasia

This form of hyperplasia is restricted to the endometrial glands and is always focal in nature, often very sharply so, hence, again, biopsy specimens may include both hyperplastic and normal endometrium. In the hyperplastic areas there is always crowding of the glands with a reduction in the amount of intervening stroma and in severe cases the glands show a 'back-to-back' pattern (Figure 9.8) with the interglandular stroma being reduced either to a thin wisp, often detectable only by

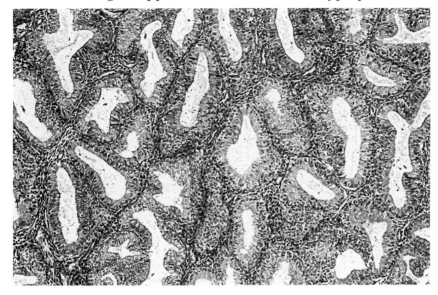

Figure 9.8 Atypical hyperplasia. Intense crowding of the glands which have assumed a 'back-to-back' pattern. The lining epithelium is stratified and exhibits a mild loss of polarity. Haematoxylin and Eosin × 93.

reticulin stains, or completely obliterated. The glands may have an outline similar to that seen in a complex hyperplasia but are usually markedly irregular in shape, showing a degree of deformity which goes beyond that explicable solely in terms of multiple outbuddings. The cells lining the hyperplastic glands tend to be larger than those seen in a normal proliferative endometrium and show varying degrees of both cytological and nuclear atypia (Figure 9.9). In the milder forms of atypical hyperplasia the nuclei are ovoid or sausage-shaped, the nucleo-cytoplasmic ratio is normal or only slightly increased, nuclear polarity is retained, the nucleoli are not enlarged and there is a normal nuclear chromatin pattern. In more severe cases of atypical hyperplasia the nucleo-cytoplasmic ratio is increased, the nuclei tend to be enlarged and rounded, nuclear polarity is disturbed or lost, nucleoli are increased in size and nuclear chromatin may be either clumped or cleared. If clearing of nuclear chromatin occurs the nuclear membrane is often very prominent. The cytoplasm may be relatively sparse in the milder forms of atypical hyperplasia but can, rather curiously, be relatively abundant in some cases of severe atypia.

There is commonly, but not invariably, some pseudostratification of the cells lining the glands in the milder forms of atypical hyperplasia and with progressing severity of the atypia there is an increasing degree of multilayering (Figure 9.10) and of intralumenal tufting and budding (Figure 9.11). In severe cases, the intralumenal tufting may be of a complex pattern and the tufts can fuse to give a cribriform pattern within the glands (Figure 9.12). These apparent intraglandular epithelial bridges retain a stromal support, albeit one which may only be revealed by a trichrome or reticulin stain. Mitotic figures are uncommon in cases of hyperplasia with mild atypia but tend to be more numerous in the more severely atypical glands, and are usually of normal form.

9.3   Interrelationships of the various forms of hyperplasia

Each form of endometrial hyperplasia has been described separately but it is not uncommon to encounter, within a single biopsy specimen, various combinations of hyperplastic patterns. Simple hyperplasia commonly exists in a pure form but it is by no means unusual to encounter a combination of simple hyperplasia with either complex or atypical hyperplasia, or both. Conversely, whilst a pure complex hyperplasia may

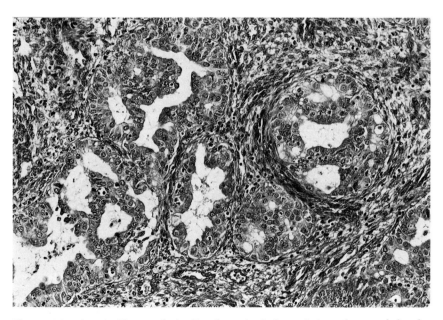

Figure 9.9   Atypical hyperplasia. Focal cytological atypia in a cluster of closely-packed glands. The glandular epithelium exhibits loss of nuclear polarity, stratification and forms bridges across the lumina. Haematoxylin and Eosin × 186.

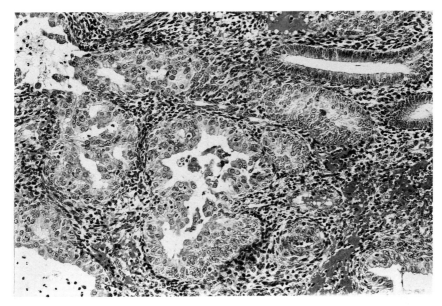

Figure 9.10 Atypical hyperplasia. The glands to the lower left of the field are lined by a stratified epithelium in which nuclear polarity is lost and in which intraluminal budding and bridging are apparent. Haematoxylin and Eosin × 186.

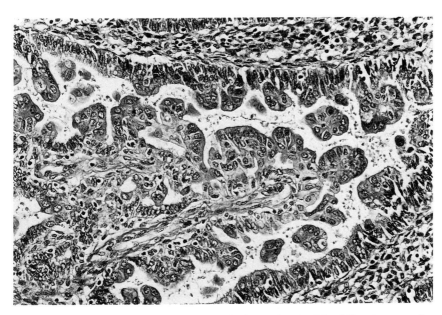

Figure 9.11 Atypical hyperplasia. Marked intraluminal budding in one of a group of glands showing atypical hyperplasia. Haematoxylin and Eosin × 232.

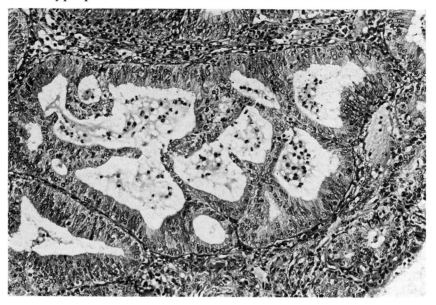

Figure 9.12 Atypical hyperplasia. The glandular epithelium forms bridges across the lumen of a gland in a focus of atypical hyperplasia. Haematoxylin and Eosin × 186.

be found in isolation there is often an accompanying simple or atypical hyperplasia. Atypical hyperplasia is commonly associated with a complex hyperplasia or, less frequently, with a simple hyperplasia.

These complicated interrelationships may suggest that the various forms of hyperplasia are either different morphological expressions of a common basic abnormality of growth or that they form a continuous spectrum. In fact there is no evidence that a simple hyperplasia is a precursor of a purely glandular hyperplasia for transitional forms between simple and glandular hyperplasia are not seen. Even when both are present in the same endometrial biopsy there is almost invariably a sharp and clear boundary between the two abnormal patterns. On the other hand a complex hyperplasia does often appear to evolve into an atypical hyperplasia and transitional stages between these two forms of glandular hyperplasia are commonly seen. However, it is not known whether a complex hyperplasia commonly, or even usually, evolves into an atypical hyperplasia.

9.4   Endometrial adenocarcinoma *in situ*

Before discussing the histological differentiation of atypical hyperplasia from an endometrial adenocarcinoma it is necessary to consider what precisely is meant in this context by the term 'adenocarcinoma'. It is perfectly clear that an adenocarcinoma which is invading the myometrium is a true malignant neoplasm but there has been considerable controversy as to the meaning of 'endometrial adenocarcinoma *in situ*'. This term has, in fact, been used in several different ways in accounts of endometrial pathology (Hertig *et al.*, 1949; Gusberg and Kaplan, 1963; Vellios, 1974). Some have equated adenocarcinoma *in situ* with severe atypical hyperplasia whilst others, though drawing a clear distinction between these two entities, have not always specified whether they consider an *in situ* adenocarcinoma one which is not invading the endometrial stroma or one which is not invading the myometrium. An adenocarcinoma *in situ* is, by presumed definition, a non-invasive lesion and therefore a true adenocarcinoma *in situ* is one in which the glands have undergone neoplastic change but in which there is no invasion of the endometrial stroma. It is debatable whether an adenocarcinoma of this type exists or if it could be recognized even if it did. Therefore a form of nomenclature has to be found to describe a lesion, which though thought to be adenocarcinomatous in nature, is confined to the endometrium and does not invade the myometrium. The term 'stage 0 carcinoma' has been applied to a lesion of this type but this is using a clinical staging system to describe a histological finding. The terms 'focal' and 'early' adenocarcinoma have little merit but the term 'intra-endometrial adenocarcinoma' seems appropriate and fully descriptive.

9.5   Histological distinction between hyperplasia and adenocarcinoma

There should not be any difficulty in distinguishing simple or complex hyperplasia from an adenocarcinoma in a curettage specimen. The differentiation in such specimens between a severe atypical hyperplasia and a well-differentiated adenocarcinoma does, however, pose a real problem which is not yet fully solved. Suggested criteria for diagnosing a neoplastic, rather than a hyperplastic, lesion include the formation of intraglandular epithelial bridges lacking any stromal support, the presence of polymorphonuclear leucocytes and nuclear debris within glandular lumens, stratification of cells to form a 'gland-within-gland' pattern, loss of nuclear polarity, marked nuclear irregularity, rounding of the nuclei, nucleolar prominence, the finding of numerous mitotic figures, the complete absence of stroma between glands, the piling up of cells into random sheets or masses, the finding of abnormal mitoses and proliferation of metaplastic squamous cells to form solid sheets which replace glands (Silverberg, 1977; Tavassoli and Kraus, 1978; Robertson, 1981; Kurman and Norris, 1982; Hendrickson *et al.*, 1983; Norris *et al.*, 1986). Features suggested as indicating stromal invasion, and therefore implying the malignant nature of the glands, include a desmoplastic reaction in the intervening stroma and focal stromal necrosis (Silverberg, 1977; King *et al.*, 1984).

In practice, many of these features appear to be of relatively little discriminatory value and it is our view that there are only a few cardinal findings in a biopsy which prompt a diagnosis of well-differentiated adenocarcinoma rather than atypical hyperplasia. These are:

i.   True intraglandular epithelial bridges which are devoid of a stromal support (Figure 9.13).

ii. The random piling up into sheets or masses of cells with rounded, irregular, usually cleared, nuclei and scanty cytoplasm (Figure 9.14).

iii. The presence of abnormal mitotic figures.

iv. The presence of polymorphonuclear leucocytes and nuclear debris within glandular lumens (Figure 9.15).

v.   Evidence of stromal invasion, i.e. stromal fibrosis, stromal necrosis, stromal polymorphonuclear leucocytic infiltration.

The pathologist should not expect all these features to be present in

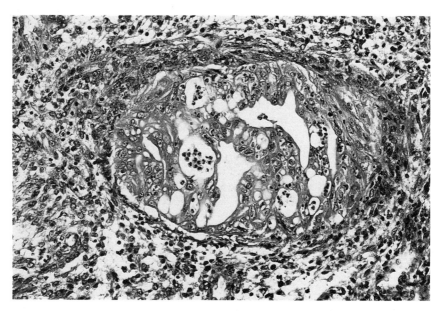

Figure 9.13 Intra-endometrial adenocarcinoma. Glandular epithelium forms disorganized proliferations and unsupported epithelial bridges within the lumen of the gland. Haematoxylin and Eosin × 232.

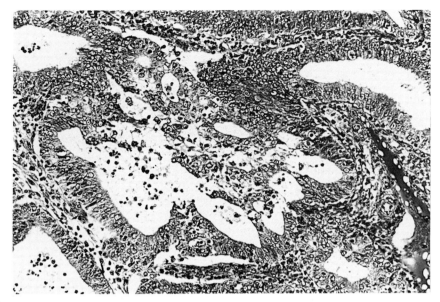

Figure 9.14 Intra-endometrial carcinoma. A further example of unsupported epithelial bridges and disorganized epithelial proliferations (epithelial anarchy). Haematoxylin and Eosin × 186.

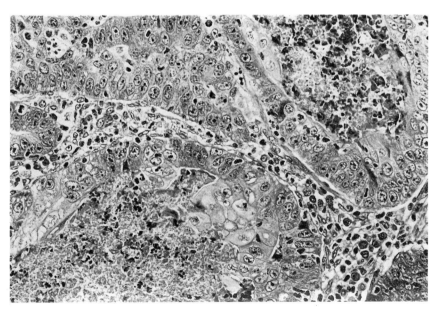

Figure 9.15 Intra-endometrial carcinoma. The glands, lined by profoundly atypical epithelium which shows abnormalities of nuclear chromatin dispersion, and contains nucleoli, are focally infiltrated by polymorphonuclear leucocytes. Haematoxylin and Eosin × 370.

biopsy material from every case of well-differentiated adenocarcinoma. Indeed, abnormal mitotic figures, perhaps the most reliable indicator of a neoplastic process, are encountered very infrequently in well-differentiated endometrial adenocarcinomas whilst it is often impossible to assess whether stromal invasion is present or not in curettings, largely because glands in such material, whether from a hyperplastic or a neoplastic process, are frequently in such close apposition that very little stromal tissue is present.

We are reasonably assured that application of the above criteria will, nevertheless, lead to an accurate differentiation between atypical hyperplasia and adenocarcinoma in the vast majority of cases. We use the term 'adenocarcinoma' in this respect to mean an endometrial neoplasm which is invading the myometrium. We are less certain that we can clearly distinguish, in biopsy material, between a severe atypical hyperplasia and an intra-endometrial adenocarcinoma; indeed, even in a hysterectomy specimen, the distinction between these two conditions is, unless stromal invasion is clearly apparent, often a matter of opinion rather than of fact.

Whilst we do think that the discriminatory criteria we utilize will exclude cases of atypical hyperplasia we recognize that they will also exclude some cases of very well-differentiated adenocarcinoma. False 'positives' and false 'negatives' are bound to occur when attempting to distinguish between atypical hyperplasia and adenocarcinoma and pathologists have to decide whether the diagnostic criteria they set are more likely to lead to an excess of false positives or to an undue number of false negatives. The natural tendency of a pathologist faced with an equivocal case is towards overdiagnosis in favour of adenocarcinoma. This attitude is spurred by the fear of 'missing' a neoplasm, exacerbated by the increasing tendency of the public to resort to litigation and has resulted, as Robertson (1981) has remarked, in the unnecessary sacrifice of many uteri on the altar of atypical hyperplasia of the endometrium. We feel, however, that diagnostic criteria should be set towards under-diagnosis, particularly in younger women. There is little, if anything, which is eventually lost, either in therapeutic or prognostic terms, by using criteria which will include a few very well-differentiated adeno-carcinomas within the diagnostic category of atypical hyperplasia and much to be gained in terms of avoidance both of unnecessary loss of reproductive capacity and of the psychological trauma of a diagnosis of cancer.

References

Fox, H. and Buckley, C.H. (1982) The endometrial hyperplasias and their relationship to endometrial neoplasia. *Histopathology*, **4**, 493–510.

Gusberg, S.B. and Kaplan, A.L. (1963) Precursors of corpus cancer. IV. Adenomatous hyperplasia as Stage 0 carcinoma of the endometrium. *Am. J. Obstet. Gynecol.*, **87**, 662–76.

Hendrickson, M.R. and Kempson, R.L. (1987) Endometrial hyperplasia and carcinoma. In *Haines and Taylor: Obstetrical and Gynaecological Pathology* (ed. H. Fox), Churchill Livingstone, Edinburgh, pp. 354–404.

Hendrickson, M.R., Ross, J.C. and Kempson, R.L. (1983) Towards the development of morphologic criteria for well-differentiated carcinoma of the endometrium. *Am. J. Surg. Pathol.*, **7**, 819–38.

Hertig, A.T., Sommers, S.C. and Bengloff, H. (1949) Genesis of endometrial carcinoma *in situ*. *Cancer*, **2**, 964–71.

King, A., Seraj, I. and Walner, R.J. (1984) Stromal invasion in endometrial adenocarcinoma. *Am. J. Obstet. Gynecol.*, **149**, 10–15.

Kurman, R.J., Katminiski, P.F. and Norris, H.J. (1985) The behaviour of endometrial hyperplasia: a long-term study of 'untreated' hyperplasia in 170 patients. *Cancer*, **56**, 403–12.

Kurman, R.J. and Norris, H.J. (1982) Evaluation of criteria for distinguishing atypical endometrial hyperplasia from well-differentiated adenocarcinoma. *Cancer*, **49**, 2547–59.

Norris, H.J., Connor, M.P. and Kurman, R.J. (1986) Preinvasive lesions of the endometrium. *Clinics Obstet. Gynaecol.*, **13**, 725–38.

Robertson, W.B. (1981) *The Endometrium*, Butterworths, London.

Silverberg, S.G. (1977) *Surgical Pathology of the Uterus*, John Wiley, New York.

Tavassoli, F. and Kraus, F.T. (1978) Endometrial lesions in uteri resected for atypical endometrial hyperplasia. *Am. J. Clin. Pathol.*, **70**, 770–79.

Vellios, F. (1974) Endometrial hyperplasia and carcinoma *in situ*. *Gynec. Oncol.*, **2**, 152–9.

Welch, W.R. and Scully, R.E. (1977) Precancerous lesions of the endometrium. *Hum. Pathol.*, **8**, 503–12.

10 Carcinoma of the endometrium (endometrial Müllerian epithelial tumours)

The pathologist dealing with a biopsy from a case of suspected carcinoma of the endometrium has first to confirm or refute the presence of a neoplasm. If a carcinoma is diagnosed the pathologist must then proceed to:

  i. Identify the precise histological type of the tumour.
 ii. Assess the grade of the tumour.
iii. Distinguish between an endocervical and an endometrial tumour.
 iv. Judge whether any non-neoplastic endometrium included in the biopsy is normally cycling, atrophic or hyperplastic.
  v. Assess, in some cases, whether fractional curettage reveals evidence of cervical involvement by an endometrial neoplasm.

The last three tasks are common to all types of endometrial carcinomas but the problem of grading differs with the histological type.

10.1 Classification of endometrial carcinomas

The histological classification of endometrial carcinomas shown in Table 10.1 is very similar to that currently recommended by the International Society of Gynecological Pathologists but differs slightly in our regarding the adenosquamous carcinoma as a discrete entity, rather than as a variant of an endometrioid adenocarcinoma, and in our recognition of the Sertoliform variant of the endometrioid adenocarcinoma.

The term 'endometrioid adenocarcinoma' merits comment. The vast majority of endometrial adenocarcinomas (80%) show some degree of endometrial differentiation and bear a resemblance, albeit an anarchic one, to normal proliferative endometrium; these are therefore 'the usual type of endometrial adenocarcinoma'. A more succinct alternative is, however, required for this unwieldy phrase and it is becoming increasingly acceptable to class such neoplasms as 'endometrioid adenocarcinomas', a term not to everyone's taste but one which is semantically, even pedantically, correct.

166

Table 10.1 Classification of primary epithelial neoplasms of the endometrium

1. Endometrioid adenocarcinoma
   Variants
       with squamous metaplasia
       papillary
       secretory
       ciliated cell
       Sertoliform
2. Adenosquamous carcinoma
3. Serous papillary adenocarcinoma
4. Clear cell adenocarcinoma
5. Mucinous adenocarcinoma
6. Squamous cell carcinoma
7. Undifferentiated carcinoma

It has to be emphasized that a simple diagnosis of 'endometrial adenocarcinoma' represents an inadequate response to the finding of a carcinoma in an endometrial biopsy. Some of the histological sub-types in Table 10.1 have a particularly poor prognosis and their identification in a diagnostic curettage is of great importance in the planning of definitive therapy.

10.2   Endometrioid adenocarcinoma

All neoplasms in this category show, by definition, some degree of endometrial differentiation. The majority are well-differentiated and consist of irregular, complex glandular acini which are lined by a predominantly cuboidal or low columnar epithelium of recognizably endometrial type (Figure 10.1). There is a marked shift, in favour of the glandular component, in the gland to stroma ratio and the glandular acini are often separated from each other only by a thin wisp of stroma or show a true 'back-to-back' pattern.

The epithelium lining the neoplastic acini shows a variable degree of multilayering and intra-acinar tufting (Figure 10.2) whilst intraglandular epithelial bridges, lacking any stromal support, are a characteristic feature and will, if widespread, impart a cribriform appearance to the neoplasm. The epithelial nuclei may be rather bland and ovoid-shaped but are more commonly rounded with either irregular, jagged condensation or a complete clearing of nuclear chromatin. Perhaps the most characteristic nuclear pattern is that of rounded nuclei with sharply etched limiting membranes and cleared chromatin. This nuclear pattern

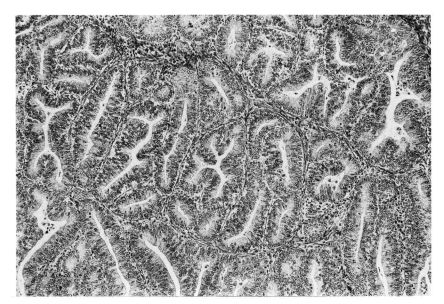

Figure 10.1 Well-differentiated endometrioid adenocarcinoma (Histological Grade 1). The tumour is composed of closely-packed, well-formed glandular acini, lined by a stratified columnar epithelium, set in a fibrous stroma. Haematoxylin and Eosin × 117.

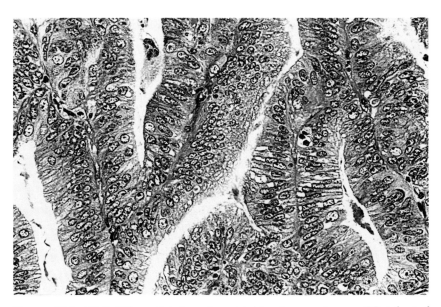

Figure 10.2 Well-differentiated endometrioid adenocarcinoma (Histological Grade 1). The glandular acini are lined by stratified columnar epithelium. The nuclei are round to oval, some contain nucleoli, and there is some loss of nuclear polarity. Note the finely dispersed nuclear chromatin in this biopsy fixed in Bouin's fixative. Haematoxylin and Eosin × 370.

can, however, be induced simply by inadequate fixation (Hendrickson and Kempson, 1987) and hence note should be taken of whether the nuclei of stromal or inflammatory cells in the biopsy specimen also show this appearance (Figure 10.3). The cleared, rounded nuclei are often aggregated into syncytial-like intra-acinar masses ('cellular anarchy') whilst mitotic figures, almost invariably of normal form, are usually present, their absence indicating considerable diagnostic caution.

Foci of necrosis are common, even in very well-differentiated tumours, and these are often infiltrated by polymorphonuclear leucocytes. Even more characteristic is the presence of such cells within glandular acini in non-necrotic areas of the tumour. The presence of foamy cells in the stroma (Figure 10.4), either singly or in clumps, is a characteristic, but by no means diagnostic, feature of endometrioid adenocarcinomas (Dalwagne and Silverberg, 1982).

A minority of endometrioid adenocarcinomas are less well-differentiated and have a partly acinar and a partly solid pattern. In such neoplasms the degree of cytological atypia is greater than in the well-differentiated tumours whilst nuclear abnormalities are more marked; mitotic figures are abundant and some will be of abnormal form.

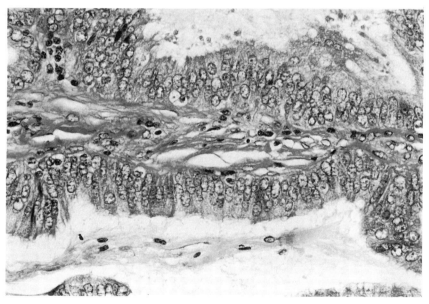

Figure 10.3   Well-differentiated endometrioid adenocarcinoma. This tumour is morphologically similar to that shown in Figure 10.2, but the tissue has been fixed more slowly in formalin. The nuclei of both the malignant epithelium and, importantly, the nuclei in the stromal cells appear 'cleared' and the nuclear membranes are therefore relatively more prominent. This is an artifact. Haematoxylin and Eosin × 370.

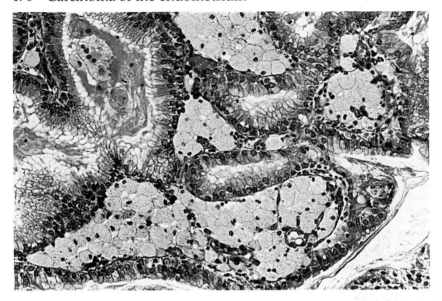

Figure 10.4 Aggregates of foamy histiocytes in the stroma of a well-differentiated endometrioid adenocarcinoma. Haematoxylin and Eosin × 232.

Poorly-differentiated endometrioid adenocarcinomas are relatively rare, have a predominantly solid growth pattern and usually show marked atypia. They can only be recognized as being of endometrioid type if there is, in some areas at least, a tentative attempt at formation of endometrial-like glandular acini.

10.2.1   Grading of endometrioid adenocarcinoma

Grading of endometrioid adenocarcinoma in curettings may, rather obviously, be less than satisfactory because of the limited sampling of the neoplasm. Nevertheless a provisional grading should be attempted because tumour grade is an important consideration when planning therapy. The traditional grading of endometrioid adenocarcinomas into well, moderately and poorly-differentiated adenocarcinomas is highly subjective and a modified FIGO grading system is recommended:

Grade I.   5% or less of the tumour shows a solid growth pattern.
Grade II.   Between 5 and 50% of the tumour is growing in a solid fashion (Figure 10.5).
Grade III.   More than 50% of the tumour shows a solid growth pattern (Figure 10.6).

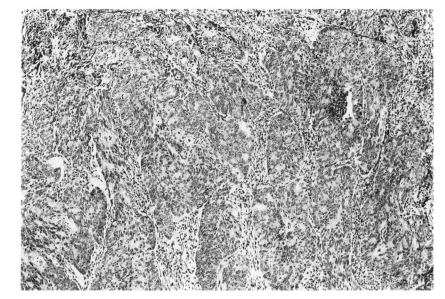

Figure 10.5 Moderately well-differentiated endometrioid adenocarcinoma (Histological Grade 2). Glandular acini are poorly formed, though approximately 50% of the neoplasm has a glandular/acinar pattern. Haematoxylin and Eosin × 93.

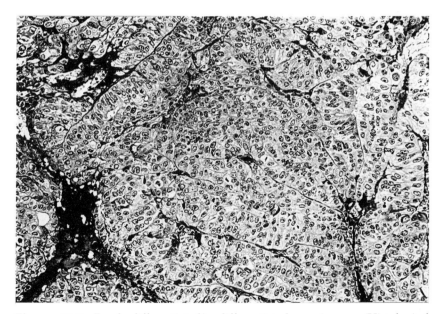

Figure 10.6 Poorly-differentiated/undifferentiated carcinoma (Histological Grade 3). The neoplasm is composed of sheets and nests of large, round to oval cells with vesicular nuclei in which there are prominent nucleoli. Haematoxylin and Eosin × 186.

In making this grading, solid sheets of cells in an endometrioid adenocarcinoma should be regarded as glandular unless definite evidence of squamous differentiation is present.

The above grading system takes account only of the architectural pattern of the tumour and neglects cytological features. In order to rectify this omission nuclear grading (Connelly et al., 1982) should also be undertaken:

Grade 1.   Oval or elongated nuclei with evenly distributed chromatin, inconspicuous nucleoli and few mitoses.

Grade 3.   Irregular rounded nuclei with prominent enlarged eosinophilic nucleoli and frequent mitoses (Figure 10.7).

Grade 2 shows features falling between Grades 1 and 3. If a carcinoma is Grade I or II on the FIGO grading system it should be raised a Grade if it shows Grade 3 nuclear abnormalities.

10.2.2   Differential diagnosis

The problem of distinguishing between a well-differentiated endometrioid adenocarcinoma and an atypical hyperplasia of the endometrium has been fully discussed in Chapter 9 and the arguments outlined there will not be repeated in this chapter.

A menstrual endometrium is sometimes misconstrued as an endometrioid adenocarcinoma but this solecism can be avoided if the disproportionate degree of haemorrhage and necrosis and, most importantly, the lack of cytological atypia in a menstrual endometrium are recognized.

A very poorly-differentiated adenocarcinoma can resemble an endometrial stromal sarcoma but a careful search for tentative gland formation, the noting of PAS positive mucus, the findings of reticulin fibres surrounding groups of cells (rather than individual cells) and the demonstration of positive staining reactions for both epithelial membrane antigen and cytokeratins and a negative reaction for vimentin will usually allow for the recognition of an adenocarcinoma. It should, however, be noted that a proportion of endometrial adenocarcinomas co-express both cytokeratins and vimentin (Dabbs et al., 1986), thus posing a diagnostic trap for those placing undue reliance on immunohistochemical techniques.

A malignant lymphoma of the endometrium can also resemble a poorly-differentiated adenocarcinoma. Lymphomas, however, often envelop normal endometrial glands, have a different nuclear pattern to that of an adenocarcinoma and are characterized by a positive staining reaction for leucocyte common antigen and a negative reaction for epithelial markers.

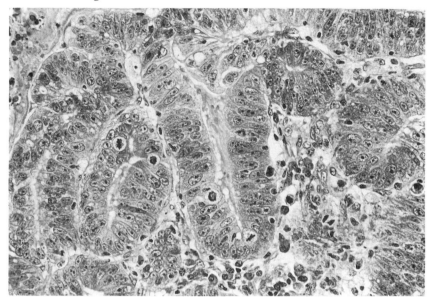

Figure 10.7 Endometrioid adenocarcinoma (Histological Grade II). Despite the presence of well-formed glandular acini, the degree of cytological atypia in this tumour is severe. Mitotic activity is prominent, nucleocytoplasmic ratios are high and there is loss of cellular polarity. Haematoxylin and Eosin × 370.

10.3   Histological variants of endometrioid adenocarcinoma

10.3.1   Endometrioid adenocarcinoma with squamous or morular metaplasia

Squamous metaplasia is very common in endometrioid adenocarcinomas and can be a conspicuous feature. It may occur as foci of bland, well-differentiated squamous tissue, as morules or as masses of keratin. Foci of well-differentiated metaplastic squamous tissue are usually clearly seen to be within neoplastic glandular acini (Figure 10.8), blend with the epithelial cells lining the acini, have a fully benign appearance and show typical squamous features, such as keratinization, intercellular bridges, sharp cell margins and eosinophilic cytoplasm; there is no invasion of the stroma by the squamous element of the tumour.

Morules (Chapter 8) consist of nests of cells, often spindly in shape, with bland, relatively small, uniform nuclei and moderately abundant, sometimes eosinophilic, cytoplasm (Hendrickson and Kempson, 1987). Occasional foci of overt squamous differentiation may be seen in some of these cell nests and large morules can, on occasion, show central necrosis. The morules lie within neoplastic acini and do not invade the stroma;

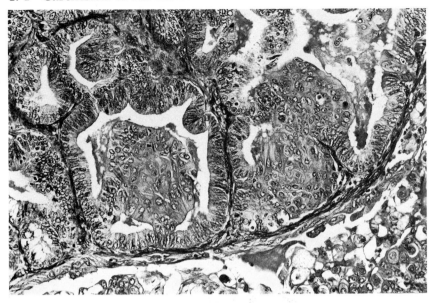

Figure 10.8 Foci of squamous metaplasia in the glandular acini of a well-differentiated endometrioid adenocarcinoma. Note that the foci of metaplastic squamous epithelium are composed of mature cells lacking cytological atypia and occupy an intraglandular site. Haematoxylin and Eosin × 232.

not uncommonly, however, the morules expand to compress, and sometimes mask or even obliterate, the surrounding glandular cells.

Squamous metaplasia in an endometrioid adenocarcinoma is occasionally manifest only by the presence of masses of keratinous tissue. These are sometimes hyalinized, may evoke a foreign body giant cell reaction (Figure 10.9) and can be so abundant as to obscure the underlying adenocarcinoma.

Endometrioid adenocarcinomas showing marked squamous metaplasia are usually Grade I and the presence of the extensive metaplastic tissue often makes the task of distinguishing in a biopsy between a complex hyperplasia and an adenocarcinoma more difficult. The principles already outlined for differentiating these two entities are not, however, altered by the presence of the metaplastic tissue.

A clear distinction has to be drawn between endometrioid adenocarcinoma showing squamous metaplasia and adenosquamous carcinomas (p. 180). Some maintain that these apparently discrete entities are just two extremes of a spectrum of increasing atypia of the squamous tissue (Hendrickson and Kempson, 1987) but it is our view that they are entirely different lesions which lack any intervening continuum. The

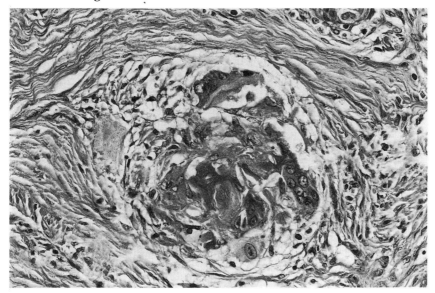

Figure 10.9   Foreign body reaction to the presence of keratin produced by an endometrioid adenocarcinoma in which there were extremely extensive foci of squamous metaplasia. The granuloma contains several macrophage giant cells surrounding irregular aggregates of keratin. Haematoxylin and Eosin × 370.

distinction between these two entities rests upon the clearly bland nature of the metaplastic squamous epithelium in an endometrioid adenocarcinoma, its lack of mitotic figures and its intraglandular non-invasive site. It is true that metaplastic squamous tissue may, on occasion, show a minor degree of atypia but this, in itself, does not justify a diagnosis of adenosquamous carcinoma.

A final problem of differential diagnosis is that morules which have obliterated the acini within which they have arisen may be regarded as solid foci of carcinoma, a mistake that can lead to inaccurate grading. Again, however, the distinction is based on the bland nature of the morules, their small uniform nuclei contrasting sharply with the large, atypical nuclei seen in solid masses of carcinomatous cells.

Endometrioid adenocarcinomas with extensive squamous metaplasia are graded only on the characteristics of the carcinomatous tissue, in exactly the same way as are similar neoplasms lacking metaplastic squamous elements and, because most endometrioid adenocarcinomas with extensive squamous metaplasia are Grade I, they generally have a good prognosis. There has been a tendency to class these neoplasms as 'adenoacanthomas' but the criteria for recognition of such a tumour, i.e.

one showing 'extensive' metaplasia, are ill-defined, imprecise and markedly subjective. It is now clear that endometrioid adenocarcinomas showing a striking degree of squamous metaplasia are associated with a prognosis that does not differ significantly from endometrioid adenocarcinomas of similar grade showing no squamous metaplasia (Barrowclough and Jaarsma, 1980). Hence there is little justification for considering the 'adenoacanthoma' as a distinct nosological entity and this diagnostic term should probably be abandoned.

10.3.2   Papillary variant of endometrioid adenocarcinoma

Many otherwise typical endometrioid adenocarcinomas of the endometrium have a papillary pattern in some areas. In a small proportion of such neoplasms this pattern predominates (Figure 10.10), tumours of this type being also known as 'villoglandular endometrioid adenocarcinomas' (Hendrickson and Kempson, 1987) and as 'well-differentiated papillary adenocarcinomas' (Chen et al., 1985). The papillae in this variant of an endometrioid adenocarcinoma are fine and non-complex with a thin fibrovascular core. The covering epithelium is formed

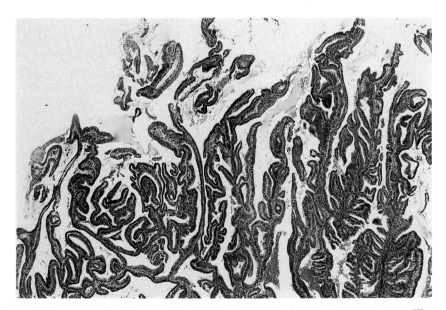

Figure 10.10 Endometrioid adenocarcinoma with papillary pattern. The superficial layers of this neoplasm are composed of fine fibrous tissue papillae covered by neoplastic epithelium. Haematoxylin and Eosin × 37.

by relatively uniform cuboidal or low columnar cells of endometrial type with ovoid, basally-situated nuclei showing only a minor degree of pleomorphism and hyperchromasia. Stratification of the covering epithelial cells is an inconspicuous feature whilst tufting is not seen. Psammoma bodies are usually absent and mitotic figures are scanty and of normal form. In most tumours of this type there is a transition, in some areas at least, to the more conventional acinar pattern of an endometrioid adenocarcinoma but this may not, of course, be apparent in a biopsy specimen.

Papillary endometrioid adenocarcinomas have an extremely good prognosis (Chen *et al.*, 1985) and it is critically important that they are distinguished from the highly aggressive serous papillary carcinoma of the endometrium (see p. 182). The distinction between these two neoplasms of vastly differing prognosis rests upon the fine nature of the papillae in the endometrioid carcinoma, on the endometrioid, rather than serous, nature of the covering epithelium and, most importantly, on the relatively low grade atypia in the epithelial cells.

10.3.3   *Secretory variant of endometrioid adenocarcinoma (Figure 10.11)*

This term is applied to those endometrioid adenocarcinomas in which the neoplastic epithelial cells show either supra- or infra-nuclear vacuolation (Tobon and Watkins, 1985); in most such neoplasms lumenal secretion is also apparent. A positive PAS staining of both the cytoplasm of the epithelial cells and the lumenal secretions, the former being rendered negative after diastase digestion, and a negative reaction with Best's carmine stain are characteristic of these neoplasms; the lumenal secretions, but not the cytoplasm of the epithelial cells, tend to stain positively with Alcian blue.

These tumours appear to be well-differentiated endometrioid adeno-carcinomas with superimposed secretory change. In premenopausal women the secretory change is probably induced by the cyclical secretion of progesterone and hence neoplasms showing a secretory pattern in curettings may not show such activity at the time of subsequent hysterectomy. In postmenopausal women the stimulus to neoplastic secretory activity is obscure if treatment with an exogenous progestagen is excluded.

Secretory endometrioid adenocarcinomas are graded in exactly the same way as are similar neoplasms lacking secretory activity and, as the vast majority are Grade I, they have a good prognosis. Secretory adenocarcinomas must, however, be distinguished from endometrial hyperplasias showing secretory change, from an Arias-Stella reaction and from a clear-cell endometrial carcinoma. The distinction of a secretory

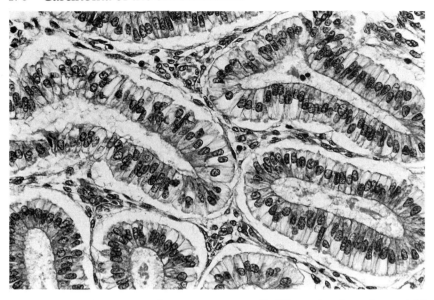

Figure 10.11 Secretory changes in a well-differentiated endometrioid adenocarcinoma. The subnuclear vacuoles seen in virtually all the epithelial cells are due to the fact that the patient had been treated with progestagens for postmenopausal bleeding. Haematoxylin and Eosin × 370.

endometrioid adenocarcinoma from hyperplasia with superimposed secretory change is based on the same principles as is the distinction between the non-secretory forms of these two entities whilst an Arias-Stella reaction can be recognized by its setting within a hypersecretory pregnancy-type endometrium. The distinction between the secretory variant of an endometrioid adenocarcinoma and the much more sinister clear cell adenocarcinoma of the endometrium (see p. 184), though not always drawn in reported series, is quite clear cut. Secretory endometrioid adenocarcinomas do not show the mixed tubulocystic, papillary and solid patterns of a clear cell adenocarcinoma, do not contain hob-nail nuclei and show a relatively minor degree of atypia.

10.3.4   Ciliated cell variant of endometrioid adenocarcinoma (Figure 10.12)

Endometrioid adenocarcinomas often contain a few ciliated cells but occasionally such neoplasms are formed predominantly, or even exclusively, of ciliated cells (Hendrickson and Kempson, 1983). These very rare tumours have a distinctive histological appearance and tend to consist of sheets of cells to which a cribriform pattern is imparted by scattered extracellular lumens. The cells limiting the lumens have

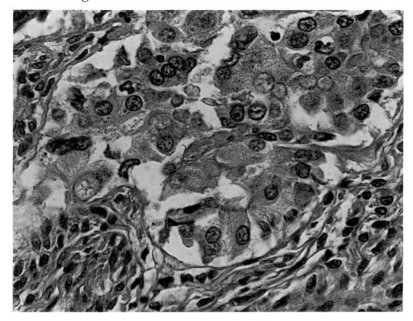

Figure 10.12   Ciliated cell carcinoma. The glandular acini are lined by cells with round to oval nuclei and copious cytoplasm. The cell surface is covered by cilia which protrude into the acinar lumen. Haematoxylin and Eosin × 575 approx. (Photograph kindly supplied by Dr R.L. Kempson.)

prominent cilia which project into the lumenal space. Many of the cells elsewhere contain sharply delineated intracytoplasmic vacuoles which contain tangled or matted eosinophilic cilia. The cells in these tumours have nuclei showing typically malignant features and, very characteristically, strongly eosinophilic cytoplasm. Many of these neoplasms contain areas of more typical endometrioid adenocarcinoma.

Grading of ciliated cell adenocarcinomas presents difficulties and it is probable that most reliance should be on nuclear, rather than architectural, grade; most are nuclear grade 1 or 2 and have a reasonably good prognosis.

It is necessary to differentiate a ciliated cell carcinoma from ciliated cell metaplasia in an endometrial hyperplasia. Again, the general principles of differentiation of a hyperplasia from an adenocarcinoma still apply.

10.3.5   Sertoliform variant of endometrioid adenocarcinoma (Figure 10.13)

Very rarely an endometrioid adenocarcinoma is composed in part of tubular structures which resemble those seen in a Sertoli cell tumour of

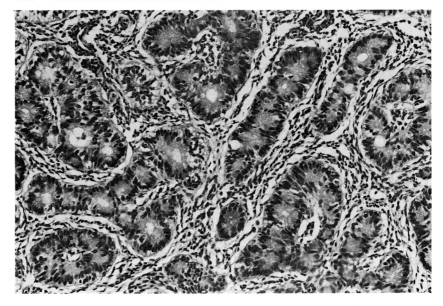

Figure 10.13 Sertoliform endometrioid adenocarcinoma. The tumour is composed of narrow, remarkably regular tubules lined by a tall columnar epithelium with well-orientated basal nuclei. There is an acute resemblance to a Sertoli cell tumour of the ovary. Elsewhere there was a transition to a more conventional endometrioid pattern. Haematoxylin and Eosin × 186.

the ovary (Fox and Brander, 1988). This should not cause confusion if, in curettage material, there is an admixture of Sertoliform tubules and conventional endometrioid adenocarcinoma. If, as could happen, the tumour tissue in a biopsy shows only a Sertoliform pattern it may be impossible to distinguish a Sertoliform adenocarcinoma from a stromal sarcoma showing a sex-cord like pattern; both lesions necessitate hysterectomy and hence an inability to make a definitive diagnosis in these circumstances is of little account.

10.4   Adenosquamous carcinoma

Tumours of this type, which account for about 5% of all endometrial neoplasms, contain both malignant glandular and malignant squamous components (Ng *et al.*, 1973; Haqqani and Fox, 1976; Alberhasky *et al.*, 1982). The glandular element of an adenosquamous carcinoma is usually an endometrioid adenocarcinoma whilst the squamous component is a squamous carcinoma of either keratinizing or non-keratinizing large cell type (Figure 10.14). In a proportion of these neoplasms the squamous

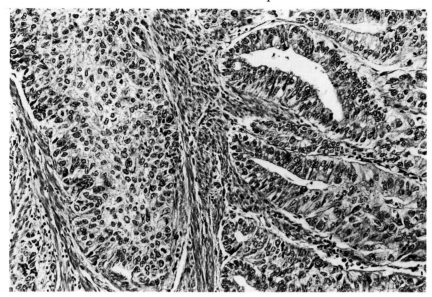

Figure 10.14   Adenosquamous carcinoma. Well-formed glandular acini lie to the right of the field and a sheet of infiltrating, non-keratinizing, large cell squamous carcinoma lies to the left. Haematoxylin and Eosin × 186.

element may show, to a variable extent, a 'glassy-cell' pattern with very distinct cell margins and eosinophilic, slightly granular cytoplasm (Christopherson *et al.*, 1982c). The squamous component may be intimately admixed with the glandular tissue but is separate from it and does not lie within glandular acini. It shows clearly malignant cytological features and infiltrates the stroma in an invasive fashion.

The appearances may be complicated by the presence of bland metaplastic squamous tissue within the acini of the adenocarcinomatous component.

Adenosquamous carcinomas are aggressive neoplasms with a relatively poor prognosis. Both components of such tumours are often present in biopsy specimens and if the biopsy contains an admixture of easily recognizable adenocarcinoma and keratinizing squamous carcinoma the distinction from the much less malignant endometrioid adenocarcinoma with squamous metaplasia is usually fairly easy, the cytologically malignant, extra-acinar, infiltrating squamous carcinoma contrasting sharply with bland, intra-acinar metaplastic squamous tissue. It is, however, necessary to ensure that these appearances are not due to a 'collision' of a cervical squamous carcinoma with an endometrial adenocarcinoma or to a cervical adenosquamous carcinoma; exclusion of these possibilities is commonly dependent on accurate clinical information.

If the squamous component of an adenosquamous carcinoma is of the non-keratinizing type it may be extremely difficult to establish its squamous nature and to distinguish it from a focus of solid adenocarcinoma. The presence of intercellular bridges and of cells with sharp margins, eosinophilic or 'glassy' cytoplasm and a relatively low nucleo-cytoplasmic ratio suggest the squamous nature of a solid group of cells whilst a P.A.S.-Alcian blue stain is useful for demonstrating a lack of mucus.

It is far from certain whether an adenosquamous carcinoma should be graded on the basis of the appearances of the glandular component, on the characteristics of the squamous component or on both. It is widely felt that only the glandular element should be graded (Hendrickson and Kempson, 1987) but it has, in fact, not been clearly established that any particular form of grading is of true prognostic value in these tumours (Christopherson, 1986). In this respect it should be noted that any difficulties encountered in differentiating sheets of non-keratinizing squamous cells from clumps of solid adenocarcinoma have little in the way of practical implications. Any endometrial carcinoma containing solid sheets of malignant cells is likely to be associated with a poor prognosis, whether these are of glandular or squamous nature.

10.5   Serous papillary carcinoma

These endometrial tumours are histologically identical to papillary serous adenocarcinomas of the ovary (Lauchlan, 1981; Christopherson et al., 1982b; Walker and Mills, 1982; Hendrickson et al., 1982; Chen et al., 1985); a current tendency to class these neoplasms as 'high grade uterine papillary carcinomas' (Hendrickson and Kempson, 1987), though correctly stressing their degree of cytological atypia, fails to identify their tubal differentiation and we therefore prefer to retain the adjective 'serous'.

Serous papillary carcinomas have, as their name indicates, a predominantly papillary architecture (Figure 10.15), sometimes simple but more commonly complex, with broad, coarse fibrovascular cores covered by pleomorphic epithelial cells; the papillary cores may be hyalinized or oedematous. The cells covering the papillae (Figure 10.16) are of serous type and show marked atypia. Their nuclei tend to be large with sharp limiting membranes, irregularly condensed chromatin and prominent eosinophilic nucleoli. The epithelial cells often show irregular pseudostratification and tufting whilst development of secondary

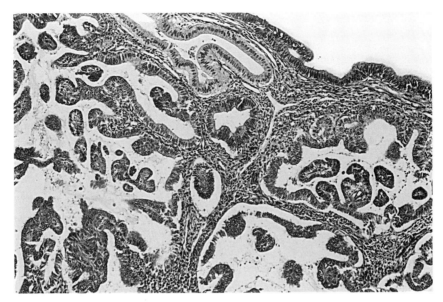

Figure 10.15 Serous papillary carcinoma. The endometrium is infiltrated by a morphologically well-differentiated papillary adenocarcinoma. Haematoxylin and Eosin × 117.

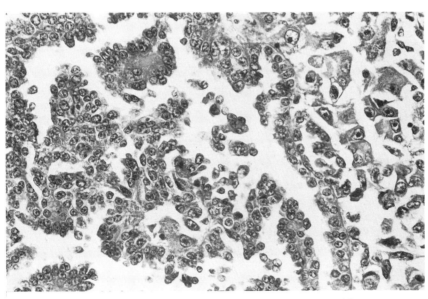

Figure 10.16 Serous papillary carcinoma. The well-formed papillary processes of the carcinoma contrast sharply with the profound cytological atypia characterized by loss of nuclear polarity, high nucleocytoplasmic ratios and, particularly in the pleomorphic cells to the right, prominent nucleoli. Haematoxylin and Eosin × 370.

papillary structures and formation of interconnecting arches are common features. Clumps of cells often exfoliate, a feature not commonly apparent in biopsy specimens, whilst mitotic figures are numerous and frequently of abnormal form. Although their architecture is generally papillary these neoplasms frequently show a solid growth pattern in some areas, with large undifferentiated cells growing in sheets which show foci of necrosis. Typical psammoma bodies are present in 30–50% of serous papillary carcinomas.

Serous papillary carcinomas of the endometrium tend to permeate, in a very extensive fashion, uterine and adnexal lymphatic and vascular channels at an early stage in their evolution and are associated with a particularly gloomy prognosis (Silverberg, 1984). It is therefore vitally important that they are distinguished from the relatively banal papillary variant of an endometrioid adenocarcinoma; the grounds for making this distinction are outlined on p. 177. A papillary serous adenocarcinoma can also resemble closely an endometrial clear cell carcinoma showing a papillary pattern but as both neoplasms share the same wretched prognosis their differentiation is of little practical importance.

Papillary serous carcinomas are graded solely on the basis of their nuclear characteristics and the vast majority are nuclear grade 2 or 3.

10.6   Clear cell adenocarcinoma

Endometrial tumours of this type are histologically identical to clear cell carcinomas of the ovary and vagina (Silverberg and DeGiorgi, 1973; Kurman and Scully, 1976; Crum and Fechner, 1979; Photopoulos *et al.*, 1979; Christopherson *et al.*, 1982a). They show a complex permutation of solid, papillary, tubulocystic and glandular patterns (Figure 10.17), though in any individual neoplasm one of these patterns may be predominantly, or even exclusively, seen. The constituent cells have abundant clear, or slightly eosinophilic, cytoplasm and large irregular nuclei with distinct, sharply angulated contours, dense chromatin and prominent nucleoli. Cells lining tubular or glandular spaces often have scanty cytoplasm and large nuclei which protrude into the lumen, the so-called 'hob-nail pattern' (Figure 10.18). In papillary areas of these neoplasms the papillae have a broad fibrovascular core and are covered by cells showing marked pleomorphism, tufting and budding. Occasional psammoma bodies may be present whilst PAS-positive diastase resistant, intracytoplasmic or intralumenal rounded bodies are frequently noted (Christopherson, 1986). The neoplasms contain abundant glycogen and, not uncommonly, a little mucus.

Clear cell adenocarcinomas are aggressive neoplasms and have a poor

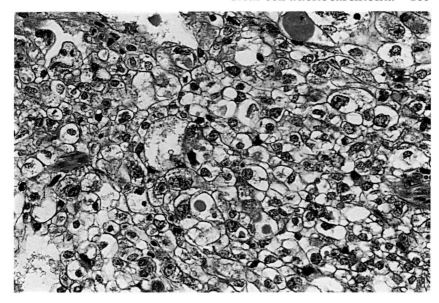

Figure 10.17 Clear cell adenocarcinoma. In this field the tumour has a solid pattern and is composed of large cells with prominent, well-defined cell margins, large nuclei and clear cytoplasm. Eosinophilic globules lie between the stromal cells. Haematoxylin and Eosin × 370.

prognosis; they can be graded only on their nuclear characteristics, though it has not been clearly shown that nuclear grading in these neoplasms correlates well with prognosis (Christopherson, 1986).

The clear cell carcinoma of the endometrium should be distinguished from an endometrioid adenocarcinoma with clear cell areas and from the secretory variant of the endometrioid adenocarcinoma. The overall architectural pattern of these two latter tumours differs considerably from that of a clear cell carcinoma whilst they show a much lesser degree of cytological and nuclear atypia. Confusion between an Arias-Stella reaction and a clear cell carcinoma can be avoided by observing the setting of the former in a typical pregnancy-type endometrium which shows no cytological atypia and by noting the lack of mitotic figures in an Arias-Stella reaction. Distinguishing between a predominantly papillary clear cell carcinoma and a serous papillary carcinoma can, especially in biopsy specimens, be a difficult and, indeed, virtually impossible, task but, as previously remarked, an inability to differentiate between these two neoplasms of similarly poor prognosis is of no practical importance. It has also to be borne in mind that a metastasis from a renal carcinoma can mimic almost exactly the appearances of a clear cell adenocarcinoma of

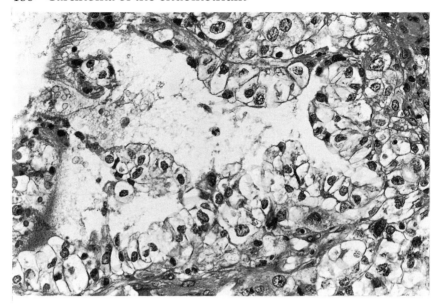

Figure 10.18   Clear cell adenocarcinoma. The glandular acini are lined by large cells with sharply defined cell margins, clear cytoplasm and prominent nuclei which, in many cells, lie at the apex of the cell, protrude into the glandular lumen and are described as having a hob-nailed appearance. Haematoxylin and Eosin × 370.

the endometrium; the only clue available for suspecting a metastasis is that renal adenocarcinomas usually show a somewhat blander nuclear pattern.

10.7   Mucinous adenocarcinoma

Many endometrioid adenocarcinomas of the endometrium contain a scattering of cells with demonstrable intracytoplasmic mucin. A small proportion of endometrial neoplasms consist predominantly of mucus-containing cells (Figure 10.19). It is suggested that the term 'mucinous adenocarcinoma' is justified when more than 50% of the cells of an endometrial adenocarcinoma contain intracytoplasmic mucin (Ross *et al.*, 1983). It should be noted that lumenal border staining for mucin, without intracytoplasmic staining, is not considered as evidence of mucinous differentiation.

Mucinous adenocarcinomas are virtually identical histologically to endocervical adenocarcinomas and to mucinous adenocarcinomas of the

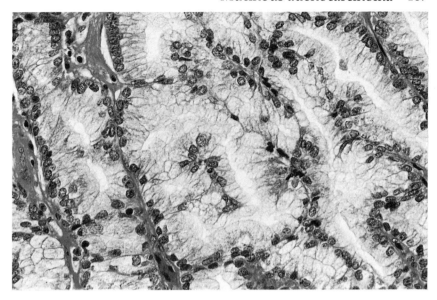

Figure 10.19 Mucinous adenocarcinoma. The glandular acini are lined by a tall mucus-secreting epithelium with well orientated basal nuclei. The absence of cytological atypia in these neoplasms may cause diagnostic problems in a small biopsy and care should be exercised in distinguishing these tumours from mucinous metaplasia. Haematoxylin and Eosin × 370.

ovary. They are usually well differentiated, show relatively mild atypia, and have a predominantly acinar pattern, though a papillary architecture is often present in some areas. The mucin, best demonstrated by PAS/ Alcian blue staining after diastase digestion, often forms intra-acinar and stromal pools which appear to attract, and are infiltrated by, poly-morphonuclear leucocytes.

Mucinous adenocarcinomas have a prognosis similar to that of endo-metrioid adenocarcinomas of the same grade and, as most are Grade I, are associated with an excellent 5-year survival rate. The often acute problem of distinguishing these adenocarcinomas from an endocervical adenocarcinoma is considered on p. 190. Mucinous adenocarcinomas have also to be differentiated from atypical endometrial hyperplasias with mucinous metaplasia, from clear cell carcinomas of the endometrium and from endometrioid adenocarcinomas with superimposed secretory change. The distinction from an atypical hyperplasia with mucinous metaplasia is based on the same general principles as that between an atypical hyperplasia and an endometrioid adenocarcinoma though it must be admitted that this task is more difficult with mucinous lesions and can, in curettage material, be almost impossible. Differentiation of a mucinous carcinoma from both a clear cell carcinoma and an endometrioid adenocarcinoma with secretory change is usually obvious on histological grounds but in occasional cases the employment of a PAS/Alcian blue stain, both before and after diastase digestion, may be helpful. As the two latter neoplasms contain an abundance of glycogen and a paucity of mucin, such findings are the reverse of those typical of a mucinous adenocarcinoma. Finally, a uterine metastasis from a colonic adenocarcinoma can be histologically identical in biopsy material, with a primary adenocarcinoma (Figure 12.7). The sharpness of this diagnostic dilemma is lessened if the adenocarcinoma is admixed with, and appears to be arising from, hyperplastic endometrium whilst a negative reaction for CEA virtually rules out the possibility of a metastasis from the colon, a positive staining reaction being however, of no discriminatory value. There are currently hopes that a monoclonal antibody which is specific for colonic neoplasms may in the future be of great diagnostic value.

10.8   Squamous cell carcinoma (Figure 10.20)

Primary squamous cell carcinomas of the endometrium are extremely rare (Lifshitz *et al.*, 1981; Yamashima and Kobara, 1986) and the belief, propagated in older reports, that they occur most commonly in elderly women with either a chronic pyometra or ichthyosis uteri seems less valid today. The finding of malignant squamous epithelium in uterine curettings will inevitably suggest that the tissue has come from a cervical squamous cell carcinoma and differentiation between a cervical and an endometrial lesion will clearly rest largely on clinical evidence. In this respect, it should be noted that a squamous cell carcinoma involving both the cervix and the endometrium is, by convention, regarded as having originated in the cervix. If a biopsy specimen showing squamous cell carcinoma is known definitely to be derived from the endometrium it is necessary to try to exclude, preferably by step-sectioning of the entire biopsy, the possibility of an adenosquamous carcinoma.

Verrucous carcinoma of the endometrium can occur (Ryder, 1982) whilst a verrucous carcinoma of the cervix may extend upwards to involve the endometrium (Tiltman and Atad, 1982). Because the diagnosis of a verrucous carcinoma rests not only on its cytological features but also on the nature of its 'pushing' base this tumour cannot be diagnosed in curettings, especially as very similar squamous tissue in endometrial biopsies may be derived from flat condylomatous lesions of the cervix which have extended into the uterine cavity (Venkatasesham and Woo, 1985; Roberts and Carrow-Brown, 1985). A squamous cell

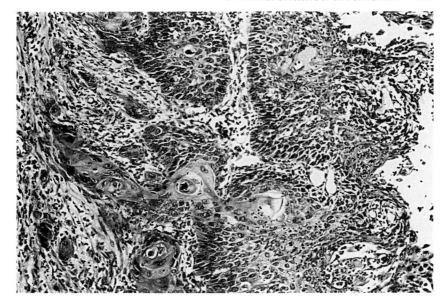

Figure 10.20 Squamous carcinoma of the endometrium. The uterus in this hysterectomy specimen is lined by squamous epithelium with features of intraepithelial neoplasia and a well-differentiated infiltrating squamous carcinoma arises from its deep surface. Haematoxylin and Eosin × 149.

carcinoma of the uterine cavity can arise from an extensive condylomatous lesion of this type.

It should be noted that cervical intra-epithelial neoplasia can also extend up into the endometrium (Salm, 1969; Kambour and Stock, 1978) and atypical epithelium of this type, covering the endometrial surface and extending into glands, may be seen in curettings.

10.9   Undifferentiated carcinoma

Undifferentiated carcinomas include, but are not limited to, giant cell, spindle cell and small cell types. Commonly the recognition of an undifferentiated carcinoma, and its distinction from a lymphoma or sarcoma, rests upon demonstration of a positive staining reaction for epithelial membrane antigen and cytokeratins and a negative reaction for leucocyte common antigen, vimentin and desmin. A particular form of undifferentiated carcinoma, the small cell carcinoma, does, however, merit special consideration. These neoplasms are identical histologically with small cell (oat cell) carcinomas of the bronchus, give a positive reaction with a Grimelius stain and are seen on electron microscopy to contain dense-core secretory granules (Paz *et al.*, 1985; Manivel *et al.*, 1986). Neoplasms of this type clearly represent a distinct nosological entity though too few have been reported for their natural history and prognosis to be clearly defined. It is important to note that argyrophil cells may be present, in small or large numbers, in any type of endometrial adenocarcinoma, the presence of such cells being of no diagnostic or prognostic importance in neoplasms other than small cell undifferentiated carcinomas (Ueda *et al.*, 1979; Bannatyne *et al.*, 1983; Sivridis *et al.*, 1984).

Undifferentiated endometrial carcinomas may show foci of multinucleated trophoblast-like differentiation (Civantos and Rywlin, 1972) and such tumours must be distinguished from a choriocarcinoma. The biphasic pattern of cytotrophoblast and syncytiotrophoblast typical of a choriocarcinoma is absent from these neoplasms whilst carcinomas showing trophoblast-like differentiation occur usually in postmenopausal patients in contrast to choriocarcinomas which arise, of course, in women of reproductive age.

10.10   Differentiation between endometrial and endocervical adenocarcinomas

In curettage material containing adenocarcinomatous tissue it may be far from clear as to whether the tumour is of endometrial or endocervical origin. This problem is at its most acute with a mucinous adenocarcinoma but can be encountered with any type of endometrial epithelial neoplasm. In many cases the clinical findings will leave little doubt as to the site of origin of the tumour whilst, in theory at least, fractional curettage should go a long way towards resolving the dilemma in clinically debatable cases. It has been our experience, however, that fractional curettage, though of diagnostic value in some cases, often yields equivocal results, thus leaving the decision as to site of origin in the hands of the pathologist.

In attempting to make a distinction between an endometrial and an endocervical neoplasm the pathologist must rely mainly on clues gleaned from a study of the non-neoplastic tissue present in the biopsy specimen. Thus, features such as a fibrotic stroma, a merging with typical endocervical epithelium or the concomitant presence of tissue showing cervical adenocarcinoma *in situ*, atypical endocervical glandular epithelium or cervical squamous intraepithelial neoplasia would all hint at an endocervical adenocarcinoma. Conversely, the presence of stromal foam cells and a merging with either normal or hyperplastic endometrium would suggest that the tumour is endometrial in nature (Hendrickson and Kempson, 1987).

It has been claimed that staining for carcinoembryonic antigen (CEA) is of some value in differential diagnosis, endocervical adenocarcinomas tending to stain positively for this antigen and endometrial tumours usually giving a negative reaction (Wahlstrom *et al.*, 1979; Ueda *et al.*, 1983). Others have, however, found a CEA stain to be of little or no discriminatory value (Cohen *et al.*, 1982; Cooper *et al.*, 1987). The use of various mucin stains to distinguish these two neoplasms also appears to be unhelpful (Hendrickson and Kempson, 1987; Cooper *et al.*, 1987).

10.11   Assessment of non-neoplastic endometrium

In curettage material containing an endometrial adenocarcinoma it is important to assess and comment upon any non-neoplastic endometrium included in the biopsy specimen. It has been clearly shown that adenocarcinomas arising from a background of atypical endometrial hyperplasia are associated with a much better 5-year survival rate than are those developing in an endometrium which is showing a normal cycling pattern, is atrophic or shows simple hyperplasia (Beckner *et al.*, 1985). Thus a comment on the characteristics of the non-neoplastic endometrium in a biopsy specimen containing endometrial adeno-carcinoma is of considerable prognostic importance.

10.12   Assessment of cervical involvement by an endometrial carcinoma

Involvement of the cervix by an endometrial adenocarcinoma will alter its stage, worsen its prognosis and demand a more aggressive therapeutic approach. Not uncommonly, therefore, endocervical curettage will be undertaken in cases of known or suspected endometrial carcinoma in order to allow assessment of cervical involvement by the pathologist. The problems involved in dealing with such biopsies have been addressed by Kadar *et al.* (1982) who recognize four different situations:

 i. The biopsy contains fragments of endometrial adenocarcinoma and of cervical tissue, these being separate from each other.
 ii. Only endometrial adenocarcinoma is present in the biopsy.
 iii. Endometrial adenocarcinoma is either replacing part of the cervical epithelium, is invading the stroma, or both.
 iv. Endometrial adenocarcinoma is infiltrating cervical stroma which is not covered by endocervical glandular epithelium.

If fragments of endometrial adenocarcinoma and cervical tissue are completely separate from each other the prognosis is the same as if endocervical curettage is negative, whilst the presence of only endometrial adenocarcinoma in curettage material cannot be taken as definite evidence of cervical involvement. The finding of endometrial adenocarcinoma infiltrating cervical stroma is clear evidence of cervical involvement but replacement of endocervical surface epithelium by endometrial adenocarcinoma is of more debatable prognostic importance. Some studies suggest that patients with this type of cervical involvement have a better prognosis than those with invasion of the cervical stroma (Kadar *et al.*, 1982).

References

Alberhasky, R.C., Connelly, P.J. and Christopherson, W.M. (1982) Carcinoma of the endometrium. IV. Mixed adenosquamous carcinoma: a clinico-pathological study of 68 cases with long-term follow-up. *Am. J. Clin. Pathol.*, **77**, 655–64.

Bannatyne, P., Russell, P. and Wills, E. (1983) Argyrophilia and endometrial carcinoma. *Int. J. Gynecol. Pathol.*, **2**, 235–54.

Barrowclough, H. and Jaarsma, K.W. (1980) Adenoacanthoma of the endometrium: a separate entity or a histological curiosity? *J. Clin. Pathol.*, **33**, 1064–7.

Beckner, M.E., Mori, I. and Silverberg, S.G. (1985) Endometrial carcinoma: nontumor factors in prognosis. *Int. J. Gynecol. Pathol.*, **4**, 131–45.

Chen, J.L., Trost, D.C. and Wilkinson, E.J. (1985) Endometrial papillary adenocarcinomas: two clinicopathological types. *Int. J. Gynecol. Pathol.*, **4**, 279–88.

Christopherson, W.M. (1986) The significance of the pathological findings in endometrial cancer. *Clinics. Obstet. Gynaecol.*, **13**, 673–93.

Christopherson, W.M., Alberhasky, R.C. and Connelly, P.J. (1982a) Carcinoma of the endometrium. I. A clinicopathologic study of clear cell carcinoma and secretory carcinoma. *Cancer*, **69**, 1511–23.

Christopherson, W.M., Alberhasky, R.C. and Connelly, P.J. (1982b) Carcinoma of the endometrium. II. Papillary adenocarcinoma: a clinical-pathological study of 46 cases. *Am. J. Clin. Pathol.*, **77**, 534–40.

Christopherson, W.M., Alberhasky, R.C. and Connelly, P.J. (1982c) Glassy cell carcinoma of the endometrium. *Hum. Pathol.*, **13**, 418–21.

Civantos, F. and Rywlin, A.M. (1972) Carcinoma with trophoblastic differentiation and secretion of chorionic gonadotrophins. *Cancer*, **29**, 789–98.

Cohen, C., Shulman, G. and Budgeon, L.R. (1982) Endocervical and endometrial adenocarcinoma: an immunoperoxidase and histochemical study. *Am. J. Surg. Pathol.*, **6**, 151–7.

Connelly, P.J., Alberhasky, R.C. and Christopherson, W.M. (1982) Carcinoma of the endometrium. III. Analysis of 865 cases of adenocarcinoma and adenoacanthoma. *Obstet. Gynecol.*, **59**, 569–75.

Cooper, P., Russell, G. and Wilson, B. (1987) Adenocarcinoma of the endocervix – a histochemical study. *Histopathology*, **11**, 1321–30.

Crum, P. and Fechner, R.E. (1979) Clear cell adenocarcinoma of the endometrium: a clinicopathologic study of 11 cases. *Am. J. Diag. Gynecol. Obstet.*, **1**, 261–7.

Dabbs, D.J., Gelsinger, K.R. and Norris, H.T. (1986) Intermediate filaments in endometrial and endocervical carcinomas: the diagnostic utility of vimentin pattern. *Am. J. Surg. Pathol.*, **10**, 568–76.

Dalwagne, M.P. and Silverberg, S.G. (1982) Foam cells in endometrial carcinoma: a clinicopathologic study. *Gynecol. Oncol.*, **13**, 67–75.

Fox, H. and Brander, S. (1988) Sertoliform adenocarcinoma of the endometrium. *Histopathology*, **13**, 584–6.

Haqqani, M.T. and Fox H. (1976) Adenosquamous carcinoma of the endometrium. *J. Clin. Pathol.*, **29**, 959–66.

Hendrickson, M. and Kempson, R.L. (1983) Ciliated carcinoma – a variant of endometrial adenocarcinoma: a report of 10 cases. *Int. J. Gynecol. Pathol.*, **2**, 13–27.

Hendrickson, M.R. and Kempson, R.L. (1987) Endometrial hyperplasia, metaplasia and carcinoma. In *Haines and Taylor: Obstetrical and Gynaecological Pathology* (ed. H. Fox), Churchill Livingstone, Edinburgh, pp. 354–404.

Hendrickson, M., Ross, J., Eiffel, P., Martinez, A. and Kempson, R. (1982) Uterine papillary serous carcinoma: a highly malignant form of endometrial carcinoma. *Am. J. Surg. Pathol.*, **6**, 93–108.

Kadar, N.R.D., Kohorn, E.I., LiVolsi, V.A. and Kapp, D.S. (1982) Histologic variants of cervical involvement by endometrial carcinoma. *Obstet. Gynecol.*, **59**, 85–92.

Kambour, A.J. and Stock, R.J. (1978) Squamous cell carcinoma *in situ* of the endometrium and Fallopian tube as superficial extension of invasive cervical carcinoma. *Cancer* **42**, 570–80.

Kurman, R.J. and Scully, R.E. (1976) Clear cell carcinoma of the endometrium: an analysis of 21 cases. *Cancer*, **37**, 872–82.

Lauchlan, S.C. (1981) Tubal (serous) carcinoma of the endometrium. *Arch. Pathol. Lab. Med.*, **105**, 615–18.

Lifshitz, S., Schauberger, C.W., Platz, C.A. and Roberts, J.A. (1981) Primary squamous cell carcinoma of the endometrium. *J. Reprod. Med.*, **26**, 25–7.

Manivel, C., Wick, M.R. and Sibley, R.K. (1986) Neuroendocrine differentiation in Müllerian neoplasms: an immunohistochemical study of a 'pure' endometrial small cell carcinoma and a mixed Müllerian tumor containing small cell carcinoma. *Am. J. Clin. Pathol.*, **86**, 438–43.

Ng, A.B.P., Reagan, J.W., Storaasli, J.P. and Wentz, W.G. (1973) Mixed adenosquamous carcinoma of the endometrium. *Am. J. Clin. Pathol.*, **59**, 765–81.

Paz, R., Frigerio, B., Sundblad, A. and Eusebi, V. (1985) Small cell (oat cell) carcinoma of the endometrium. *Arch. Pathol. Lab. Med.*, **109**, 270–72.

Photopoulos, G.J., Carney, C.N., Edelman, D.A., Hughes, R.R., Fowler, W.C. and Walton, R.A. (1979) Clear cell carcinoma of the endometrium. *Cancer*, **43**, 1448–56.

Roberts, P.F. and Carrow-Brown, J. (1985) Condylomatous atypia of the endometrial cavity. *Br. J. Obstet. Gynaecol.*, **42**, 535–8.

Ross, J.C., Eifel, P.J., Cox, R.S., Kempson, R.L. and Hendrickson, M.R. (1983) Primary mucinous adenocarcinoma of the endometrium: a clinicopathologic and histochemical study. *Am. J. Surg. Pathol.*, **7**, 715–29.

Ryder, D.A. (1982) Verrucous carcinoma of the endometrium: a unique neoplasm with long survival. *Obstet. Gynecol.*, **59**, 78s–80s.

Salm, R. (1969) Superficial intra-uterine spread of intra-epithelial cervical carcinoma. *J. Pathol.*, **97**, 261–8.

Silverberg, S.G. (1984) New aspects of endometrial carcinoma. *Clinics. Obstet. Gynacol.*, **11**, 189–208.

Silverberg, S.G. and DeGiorgi, L.S. (1973) Clear cell carcinoma of the endometrium: clinical, pathologic and ultrastructural findings. *Cancer*, **31**, 1127–40.

Sivridis, E., Buckley, C.H. and Fox, H. (1984) Argyrophil cells in normal, hyperplastic and neoplastic endometrium. *J. Clin. Pathol.*, **27**, 378–81.

Tiltman, A.J. and Atad, J. (1982) Verrucous carcinoma of the cervix with endometrial involvement. *Int. J. Gynecol. Pathol.*, **1**, 221–6.

Tobon, H. and Watkins, G.J. (1985) Secretory adenocarcinoma of the endometrium. *Int. J. Gynecol. Pathol.*, **4**, 328–35.

Ueda, G., Yamasaki, M., Indue, M. and Kurachi, K. (1979) A clinicopathologic study of endometrial carcinomas with argyrophil cells. *Gynecol. Oncol.*, **7**, 223–32.

Ueda, S., Tsubara, A., Izumi, H., Sasaki, M. and Morii, S. (1983) Immuno-histochemical studies of carcinoembryonic antigen in adenocarcinoma of the uterus. *Acta. Pathol. Jap.*, **33**, 59–69.

Venkatasesham, V.S. and Woo, T.H. (1985) Diffuse viral papillomatosis (condyloma) of the uterine cavity. *Int. J. Gynecol. Pathol.*, **4**, 370–77.

Wahlstrom, I., Lindgren, J., Korhonen, M. and Seppala, M. (1979) Distinction between endocervical and endometrial adenocarcinoma with immuno-peroxidase staining of carcinoembryonic antigen in routine histological tissue specimens. *Lancet*, **ii**, 1159–60.

Walker, A.N. and Mills, S.E. (1982) Serous papillary carcinoma of the endometrium: a clinicopathologic study of 11 cases. *Diag. Gynecol. Obstet.*, **4**, 261–7.

Yamashima, M. and Kobara, T.Y. (1986) Primary squamous cell carcinoma with its spindle cell variant in the endometrium: a case report and review of the literature. *Cancer*, **57**, 340–45.

11 Non-epithelial and mixed endometrial tumours of Müllerian origin

Endometrial stem cells of Müllerian origin have a potentiality to differentiate into epithelial cells, mesenchymal cells or both. Tumours derived from such cells may therefore be purely epithelial, solely non-epithelial or mixed. Furthermore, cells developing along a non-epithelial pathway may differentiate not only into endometrial stromal cells but also into mesenchymal elements not normally found in the uterus, such as cartilage, bone or striated muscle.

Non-epithelial endometrial neoplasms of Müllerian origin are therefore categorized either as pure, containing only non-epithelial cells, or mixed, containing both non-epithelial and epithelial components. The tumours are further subdivided on the basis of whether they consist only of homologous components, i.e. those normally present in the uterus, or whether they contain, or consist solely of, heterologous tissues which are normally alien to the uterus. A full classification of these neoplasms is given in Table 11.1. This may, at first sight, appear complex but is, if the above comments are taken into account, both logical and simple. All these neoplasms are, with the exception of leiomyomas, uncommon, the ones encountered least infrequently being the endometrial stromal sarcomas and the carcinosarcomas.

It will be appreciated that the classification shown in Table 11.1 refers only to tumours thought to be of Müllerian origin. It is possible for non-epithelial neoplasms to arise also from non-Müllerian tissues such as the blood vessels or neural elements and these rare tumours are considered in Chapter 12.

11.1 Pure non-epithelial neoplasms of endometrial stromal type

(Endometrial stromal nodule, endometrial stromal sarcomas of low and high grade malignancy.)

195

Table 11.1 Classification of uterine non-epithelial and mixed epithelial/non-epithelial tumours of Müllerian origin

---

Non-epithelial tumours
  (i) *Homologous*
      (a) Of endometrial stromal type
            Stromal nodule
            Low grade endometrial stromal sarcoma
            High grade endometrial stromal sarcoma
      (b) Of smooth muscle type
            Leiomyoma
            Leiomyosarcoma
 (ii) *Heterologous*
            Rhabdomyosarcoma
            Chondrosarcoma
            Osteosarcoma

Mixed tumours
  (i) *Homologous*
      Benign
        Adenofibroma
      Of low grade malignancy
        Adenosarcoma
        Carcinofibroma
      Of high grade malignancy
        Carcinosarcoma
 (ii) *Hetrologous*
      Of low grade malignancy
        Adenosarcoma with heterologous components
      Of high grade malignancy
        Carcinosarcoma with heterologous elements

11.1.1   Histological features

All pure endometrial stromal neoplasms have certain characteristics in common: they are formed of cells which, to a greater or lesser degree, resemble the stromal cells of the normal endometrium during the proliferative phase of the cycle, have a rich vascular supply and, by definition, lack heterologous components and epithelial elements.

The endometrial stromal nodule (Figure 11.1) is a well-circumscribed benign lesion (Norris and Taylor, 1966a; Tavassoli and Norris, 1981) whilst the endometrial stromal sarcoma of low grade malignancy (previously known either as 'uterine stromatosis' or as 'endolymphatic stromal myosis') is an infiltrative neoplasm which tends to invade blood vessels and pursue an indolently malignant course (Baggish and Woodruff, 1972; Hart and Yoonessi, 1977; Hendrickson and Kempson,

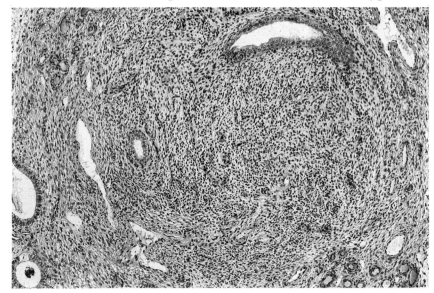

Figure 11.1 Stromal nodule. A discrete nodule of stromal cells occupies the centre of the field. There is a minor degree of glandular distortion which is the consequence of its presence but no evidence of cytological atypia or mitotic activity. Haematoxylin and Eosin × 93.

1980; Kempson and Hendrickson, 1987). A distinction between these two neoplasms rests solely on whether the tumour margin is smooth and pushing or is infiltrating and hence can only be made on examination of a hysterectomy specimen. The biopsy appearances of the two lesions are identical and they can *not* be distinguished in curettage material. Both are formed of sheets of generally uniform cells with darkly-staining, small, round or ovoid nuclei, scanty cytoplasm and ill-defined limiting membranes (Figure 11.2). Occasional cells may have fusiform nuclei and in rare instances this pattern predominates. Nuclear pleomorphism and cytological atypia are absent or minimal, necrosis is rarely seen and, by definition, there are less than 10 mitotic figures per 10 high power fields (Hendrickson and Kempson, 1980; Fekete and Vellios, 1984; Kempson and Hendrickson, 1987), these being invariably of normal form. Focal hyaline change is common and is sometimes a prominent feature with extensive areas of hyalinized tissue compressing the tumour cells into trabeculae or cords. There is a rich, ramifying vascular framework within these neoplasms, the vessels sometimes resembling spiral arterioles (Figure 11.3). A reticulin stain is of considerable value for revealing the abundance of the vasculature. Not infrequently, the tumour cells

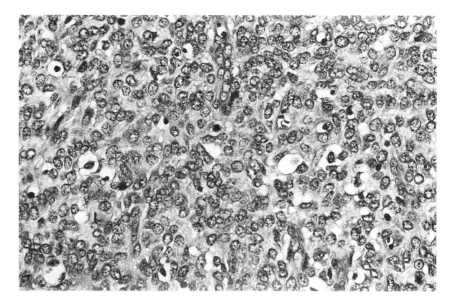

Figure 11.2 Low grade stromal sarcoma. The neoplasm is composed of sheets of cells similar to those of proliferative endometrium. There is no significant cytological atypia and mitotic activity is sparse. Haematoxylin and Eosin × 370.

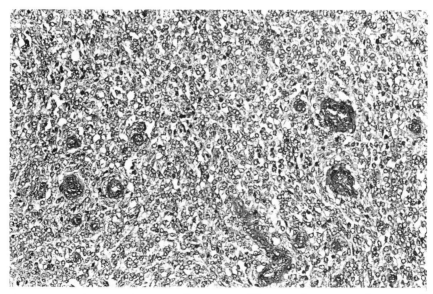

Figure 11.3 Low grade stromal sarcoma. The neoplasms are always well supplied with small blood vessels but, as in this example, they are sometimes particularly prominent. Note that they are narrow and relatively uniform in contrast to the thin-walled branching vessels of the haemangiopericytoma (Figure 12.1). Haematoxylin and Eosin × 186.

condense around the blood vessels and in the 'pericytic' variant of the low grade endometrial stromal sarcoma there is an exaggeration of this perivascular pattern.

Endometrial stromal sarcomas of high grade malignancy are extremely aggressive neoplasms which commonly lead to death within two years (Yoonessi and Hart, 1977; Fekete and Vellios, 1984; Kempson and Hendrickson, 1987). The defining feature of these neoplasms, and one which is independent of any other cytological features, is that they have more than 10 mitotic figures per 10 high power fields. These tumours may in fact only differ from stromal sarcomas of low grade malignancy in their higher content of mitotic figures but most show a much greater degree of pleomorphism and atypia than do neoplasms of lesser malignancy (Figure 11.4). Hyaline change and a pericytic pattern are rarely seen whilst, by contrast, necrosis may be a conspicuous feature. The typical vascular pattern of an endometrial stromal tumour is often lacking: indeed many neoplasms categorized as high grade stromal sarcomas lack any resemblance to endometrial stroma and would be better described as undifferentiated sarcomas.

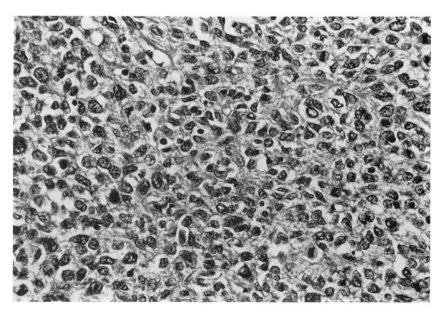

Figure 11.4   High grade stromal sarcoma with an epithelioid pattern. There is greater cytological atypia than in the low grade stromal sarcoma, the cells are more pleomorphic and mitoses are more frequent. Haematoxylin and Eosin × 370.

All cases of possible endometrial stromal neoplasm should be stained for reticulin for they demonstrate a very characteristic pattern of reticulin fibres surrounding individual cells or, at the most, small groups of cells. A PAS stain is also mandatory and will show that stromal tumours are devoid of both glycogen and mucus. Immunocytochemical stains reveal a somewhat confusing pattern for these tumours not only stain positively, as would be expected, for vimentin but also for desmin, actin, myosin, alpha-1-antitrypsin and alpha-1-chymotrypsin (Bonazzi del Poggetto *et al.*, 1983; Marshall and Braye, 1985).

11.1.2   *Differential diagnosis*

In curettage material it is necessary to differentiate stromal neoplasms from other diffuse small cell lesions. This problem arises most acutely in those endometrial stromal sarcomas of high grade malignancy which lack a typical vascular framework. Such tumours can closely resemble an anaplastic endometrial carcinoma, malignant lymphoma or leukaemic infiltration of the endometrium and, perhaps suprisingly, a severe chronic endometritis. The finding of tentative attempts at glandular differentiation, of PAS-positive mucus, of reticulin fibres surrounding alveolar masses of cells and of a positive staining reaction for common epithelial membrane antigen and cytokeratin together with a negative stain for vimentin will all favour a diagnosis of adenocarcinoma rather than endometrial stromal sarcoma. Malignant lymphoma and leukaemic infiltrates commonly tend to surround and include normal endometrial glands and are often of recognizably histiocytic or granulocytic nature. In doubtful cases the demonstration of non-specific esterase, common leucocyte antigen or B- and T-cell markers may be of diagnostic value. A very severe endometritis, of the type sometimes seen in chlamydial infections (Chapter 7) can evoke a diffuse cellular infiltrate which destroys endometrial glands and is sufficiently dense as to suggest a neoplastic process. The inflammatory nature of the infiltrate is usually revealed by the presence of ill-formed germinal centres, by the finding of tangible body macrophages and by the recognition of the lympho-plasmocytic nature of the cellular infiltrate.

The relatively few endometrial stromal sarcomas with predominantly fusiform nuclei can be confused with a leiomyosarcoma, though in most such neoplasms there is usually a transition, in at least some areas of the tumour, to a more characteristic rounded nuclear pattern. The cells in a leiomyosarcoma have more abundant cytoplasm than do those of an endometrial stromal sarcoma, a distinction made more clear with a trichrome stain, and, after staining with P.T.A.H., may be shown to contain demonstrable myofibrils. Immunocytochemical stains are of value in distinguishing between malignant smooth muscle and endometrial stromal neoplasms in so far as while both stain positively for desmin and vimentin only the latter give a positive reaction for alpha-1-antitrypsin, though admittedly not in all cases.

Endometrial stromal sarcomas of low grade malignancy, particularly those showing a pericytic pattern, may closely resemble a haemangio-pericytoma. There are many who will dispute that this presents a diagnostic problem, claiming that all apparent uterine haemangio-pericytomas are incorrectly diagnosed endometrial stromal sarcomas. We agree, however, with those who maintain that uterine haemangio-pericytomas are a genuine entity and believe that such neoplasms can usually be recognized by their content of branching, 'stag-horn' vessels (Chapter 12).

11.1.3 Differentiation between pure and mixed stromal neoplasms

There is no real possibility of confusing a pure stromal neoplasm with a typical carcinosarcoma but if a stromal sarcoma envelops and includes non-neoplastic endometrial glands a resemblance to an adenosarcoma may result. This only poses a problem in biopsy material for in hysterectomy specimens it is usually apparent that the entrapped glands are confined to the periphery or base of the tumour. This topographical aid to differential diagnosis is not discernible in a biopsy specimen in which it will nevertheless be clear that a characteristic feature of an adenosarcoma, namely condensation of neoplastic stromal cells around the glands to form a cambium layer, is absent.

Occasionally, a minor degree of glandular differentiation is apparent within an otherwise typical pure stromal neoplasm. Such glandular elements are, however, poorly formed, few and inconspicuous and their presence does not justify a diagnosis of a mixed neoplasm (Kempson and Hendrickson, 1987).

11.1.4 Assessment of degree of malignancy

It is important to assess the degree of malignancy in a stromal neoplasm diagnosed on biopsy for such a grading may well influence the nature of the subsequent surgical treatment. As already remarked the distinction in biopsy specimens is solely between tumours of high grade malignancy and neoplasms of lesser malignancy, it not being possible to draw a distinction between benign lesions and tumours of low grade malignancy. The grading of stromal tumours as being of high grade malignancy rests principally, though not solely, on their content of 10 or more mitotic figures per 10 high power fields. Mitotic counts tend to be highly subjective for mitotic figures are easily confused with lymphocytes, naked nuclei, degenerate cells or precipitated haematoxylin (Norris, 1976; Scully, 1976; Kempson, 1976; Silverberg, 1976; Ellis and Whitehead, 1981). It is necessary therefore to insist upon strict criteria for the recognition of mitotic figures and to define the technique of counting such figures in rigid terms. Hendrickson and Kempson (1980) maintain that mitotic figures should only be diagnosed if there is separation of chromatin in a cell with clear or eosinophilic cytoplasm and distinct cell membranes. We tend to follow the advice of Park (1980) who maintained that a mitotic figure should only be diagnosed as such if the pathologist is prepared to photograph it to illustrate mitosis in a student textbook.

Mitotic counts should only be performed on thin, well-stained sections which are examined in a binocular microscope using a ×10 eyepiece and a ×40 dry objective. The count has to be carried out in an obsessional manner, beginning in those areas showing the highest mitotic activity, and should consist of four sets of 10 high power fields per section, the highest count being recorded. Mitotic counts performed in this fashion give reasonably reproducible results with degrees of interobserver variation being unlikely to be of sufficient magnitude to lead to major diagnostic errors (Zaloudek and Norris, 1981a; Kempson, 1976). An alternative approach to the recording of mitotic figures is to count the number of mitoses per mm^2 of tissue (Fortune and Östör, 1987). This method takes into account the fact that even when using objective and eyepiece lenses of agreed magnification the size of a high power field will still vary with different microscopes, being influenced by such factors as the use of an intermediate lens and the field of view index. This technique of mitotic counting has much to recommend it though it has not yet achieved wide usage.

In the vast majority of pure stromal neoplasms mitotic counts yield clear-cut results, tumours of low grade malignancy usually containing less than 4 mitotic figures per 10 high power fields and neoplasms of high grade malignancy having mitotic counts well in excess of 20 per 10 high power fields. Very occasional cases will be encountered where the mitotic count is neither very low nor unduly high, i.e. 9 mitoses per 10 high power fields. In such equivocal cases account must be taken of other features of the neoplasm, such as the degree of pleomorphism and atypia, the presence of abnormal mitotic figures and the noting of areas of necrosis.

11.1.5   Endometrial tumours with a sex cord stromal pattern

Some endometrial stromal tumours, of any degree of malignancy, contain epithelial-like elements arranged in trabecular cords, nests or tubules

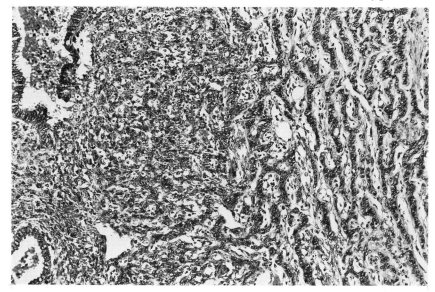

Figure 11.5 Stromal sarcoma with sex cord pattern. The endometrium is infiltrated by a low grade stromal sarcoma in which the tumour cells form well-ordered trabeculae resembling those seen in sex cord tumours of the ovary. Haematoxylin and Eosin × 149.

(Figure 11.5) and in occasional neoplasms this pattern is the predominant, or even the sole, feature. Such tumours bear a quite striking similarity to an ovarian sex cord stromal neoplasm (Clement and Scully, 1976) and can cause considerable confusion when encountered in curettage material. True sex cord stromal tumours do not occur in the uterus and the differential diagnosis (discussed in Chapter 10) is from the very rare Sertoliform endometrioid adenocarcinoma of the endometrium.

11.2   Pure non-epithelial neoplasms of smooth muscle type

Pure smooth muscle tumours of the uterus are considered here largely for the sake of completeness, for being of myometrial rather than endometrial origin they lie outside the scope of this book. Those wishing for a detailed discussion and analysis of these neoplasms are referred to Kempson and Hendrickson (1987).

Despite the above avowal, smooth muscle neoplasms can be encountered in curettage material, albeit rather uncommonly. Tissue may be obtained from a submucous leiomyoma, especially one that is polypoid, whilst it is far from unusual for a leiomyosarcoma to ulcerate through the endometrium and grow into the uterine cavity. Recognition of a leiomyomatous or leiomyosarcomatous neoplasm in a biopsy rests upon finding evidence of smooth muscle differentiation. Most leiomyomas show evident smooth muscle differentiation, being composed of elongated cells with abundant eosinophilic cytoplasm and bland cigar-shaped nuclei. Longitudinal myofibrils may be clearly seen in haematoxylin and eosin stained sections and are, in equivocal cases, more readily recognized in P.T.A.H. stained sections. A minority of leiomyosarcomas show equally clear evidence of smooth muscle differentiation but many, at the other end of the spectrum, are very poorly differentiated and are formed of a mixture of spindle and polygonal cells which lack any obvious myofibrils.

Smooth muscle neoplasms of the uterus fall into one of three categories: benign, of uncertain malignant potential and malignant. Placement of a particular neoplasm into one of these groups depends upon a consideration of the histological pattern, the degree of cellularity, the amount of atypia and the number of mitotic figures. It is important when analysing a smooth muscle neoplasm to take all these factors into account and not to rely on one finding and neglect the others.

Cellular, epithelioid, bizarre ('symplastic') and neurilemmoma-like variants of the usual leiomyoma may all be encountered in biopsies and for each of these histological types the criteria for categorization as malignant vary (Kempson and Hendrickson, 1987). Recognition of a neoplasm showing overtly sarcomatous features, such as marked atypia and a high content of mitotic figures, as malignant is obviously easy but some leiomyosarcomas are diagnosed principally, though never entirely, on mitotic counts; the technique of performing, and the inherent pitfalls in, mitotic counts have already been considered (p. 202).

In curettage material the only real problem in differential diagnosis presented by smooth muscle tumours is the distinction of poorly-differentiated leiomyosarcomas from endometrial stromal sarcomas of high grade malignancy and from poorly-differentiated endometrial carcinomas. The distinction of a leiomyosarcoma from a stromal sarcoma of high grade malignancy has already been discussed (p. 200) whilst a combination of a PAS stain, a stain for reticulin fibres and immunocytochemical stains for epithelial membrane antigen, vimentin and desmin will usually allow for a distinction to be drawn between poorly-differentiated leiomyosarcomas and carcinomas (Figure 11.6). It should be noted that a proportion of leiomyosarcomas also give a positive staining reaction for cytokeratins (Brown et al., 1987; Norton et al., 1987). This apparently paradoxical finding should not be allowed to detract from a diagnosis of leiomyosarcoma.

A final point to consider is that leiomyosarcomatous tissue in a curetting could come from either a pure neoplasm or from a mixed

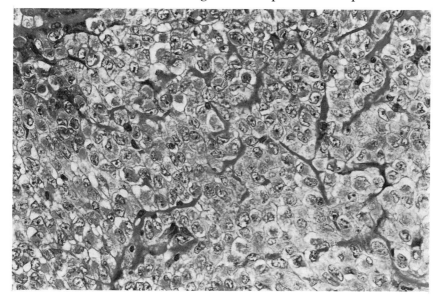

Figure 11.6   Undifferentiated sarcoma. The tumour cells have an epithelioid appearance. At the subsequent hysterectomy both leiomyomatous and rhabdomyomatous elements were identified. Haematoxylin and Eosin × 370.

Müllerian tumour. It may be impossible to decide between these two possibilities in a biopsy specimen and, as both conditions necessitate a hysterectomy, it is fruitless to worry over this diagnostic dilemma.

11.3   Pure heterologous non-epithelial neoplasms

These are extremely rare and generally take the form of a rhabdomyosarcoma (Donkers *et al.*, 1972; Hart and Craig, 1978; Vakiani *et al.*, 1982; Siegal *et al.*, 1983), osteosarcoma (Crum *et al.*, 1980) or chondrosarcoma (Clement, 1978). Rhabdomyosarcomas tend to be of the pleomorphic variety (Figure 11.7) and the histological features of all these neoplasms are identical to those of their counterparts arising in more conventional sites: they are usually clearly malignant with considerable pleomorphism, atypia and mitotic activity.

When encountered in biopsy material it is usually not possible to tell if material from a heterologous sarcoma is in fact from a pure neoplasm or is part of the mesenchymal component of a mixed Müllerian tumour of high grade malignancy. A heterologous sarcoma that has enveloped normal endometrial glands may be confused with an adenosarcoma but in such a

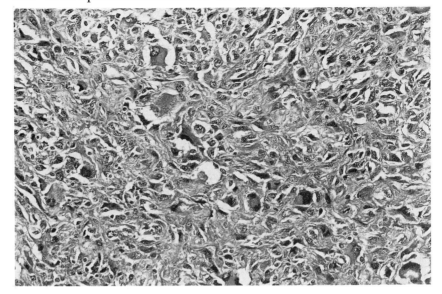

Figure 11.7   Rhabdomyosarcoma. The tumour is composed of pleomorphic cells some of which are very large and have copious eosinophilic cytoplasm with one or more eccentrically placed nucleus. Haematoxylin and Eosin × 186.

neoplasm there will not be the characteristic condensation around the included glands to form a cambium layer.

In practice, the drawing of a distinction between a pure heterologous sarcoma and a mixed tumour is of no importance for both lesions necessitate hysterectomy. It is, however, crucially important not to confuse osseous or cartilaginous metaplasia in the endometrial stroma with an osteosarcoma or a chondrosarcoma. Usually, the clearly malignant nature of the sarcomatous neoplasm contrasts sharply with the benign pattern shown by metaplastic cartilage or bone. Furthermore it can often be seen, even in biopsy material, that the metaplastic tissue is arising from, and blends smoothly with, normal endometrial stroma. Fetal remnants may also enter into the differential diagnosis of an osteosarcoma or a chondrosarcoma. Any retained fetal bone or cartilage is lacking in malignant features and is often admixed with other fetal elements, such as neural tissue (Chapter 8).

11.4   Mixed tumours

Mixed tumours contain both epithelial and non-epithelial elements, both of which may be benign (adenofibroma) or both of which may be malignant (carcinosarcoma). Between these two extremes are those neoplasms in which either the mesenchymal element is malignant and the epithelial component benign (adenosarcoma) or the epithelial element is malignant and the stromal component benign (carcinofibroma), both these latter neoplasms being grouped together as mixed tumours of low grade malignancy (Östör and Fortune, 1980; Fortune and Östör, 1987).

Mixed tumours can occur at any age but develop most frequently in postmenopausal women. They commonly form bulky polypoid masses which fill the uterine cavity and may project through the cervical os. The patients usually present with a complaint of vaginal bleeding though sometimes a vaginal discharge or the passage of tissue fragments *per vaginum* is noted.

11.4.1 Histological features

Adenofibromas (Figure 11.8) contain an admixture of benign mesenchymal and epithelial components (Vellios *et al.*, 1973; Grimalt *et*

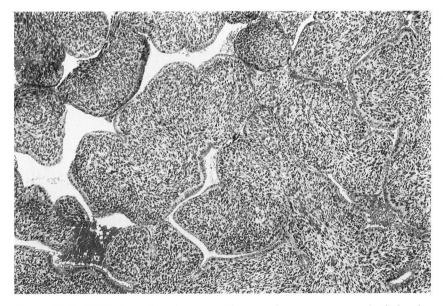

Figure 11.8 Müllerian adenofibroma. The neoplasm is composed of closely-packed, somewhat moulded, coarse papillae with fibrous tissue and endometrial stromal cores covered by a cubo-columnar epithelium of endometrial type. There is a minor degree of stromal condensation deep to the surface epithelium but it is less marked than in an adenosarcoma (Figures 11.10 to 11.12). Haematoxylin and Eosin × 93.

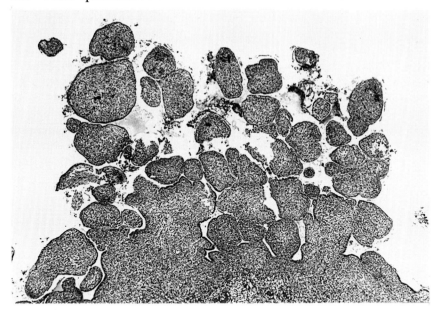

Figure 11.9 Müllerian adenofibroma. The surface of the neoplasm has a prominent papillary pattern, the papillae being covered most commonly by endometrioid epithelium or flattened epithelium of indeterminate type. Haematoxylin and Eosin × 37.

al., 1975). The epithelial element covers broad papillary fronds which project both from the surface (Figure 11.9) and into cystic spaces within the neoplasm and also forms a lining to glandular acini, clefts and cysts which are set in the mesenchymal component. The epithelial cells are cytologically bland and may be of endometrial, tubal, endocervical, squamous or nondescript cuboidal type. In many adenofibromas there is a melange of different epithelia but in some only one type, usually an endometrioid epithelium, is present. The mesenchymal component of an adenofibroma consists of endometrial-stromal-like cells, fusiform cells or a mixture of these two components. The mesenchymal tissue tends to be condensed around or beneath the epithelial component, is histologically benign, does not contain heterologous components and has a mitotic count of less than 4 per 10 high power fields (Mills *et al.*, 1981; Zaloudek and Norris, 1981b; Fortune and Östör, 1987).

The adenosarcoma contains a benign epithelial element and a malignant mesenchymal component (Clement and Scully, 1974; Fox *et al.*, 1979; Östör and Fortune, 1980; Martinelli *et al.*, 1980; Zaloudek and Norris, 1981b; Chen, 1985). At first sight these neoplasms closely resemble an adenofibroma with an epithelial component covering papillae on the surface, within clefts and lining cysts or glands embedded in the stroma (Figure 11.10). The epithelium may be of any Müllerian type as in the adenofibroma, but the most common pattern is for it to be predominantly endometrioid with a minor admixture of endocervical and squamous elements. The epithelium may show a minor degree of multilayering and irregularity but true cytological atypia is not seen. The mesenchymal component of these neoplasms tends to be predominant and is usually formed by cells with round, ovoid or fusiform nuclei, scanty cytoplasm and indistinct margins (Figure 11.11), the appearances resembling closely those of an endometrial stromal sarcoma or, less commonly, the features are those of an undifferentiated sarcoma. The sarcomatous tissue tends to be of variable cellularity and compactness but is, characteristically, condensed beneath the surface epithelium and around the contained glands or cysts (Figure 11.12) to form a distinct 'cambium' layer. Heterologous elements, such as rhabdomyoblasts, cartilage or fat, may be present in the stroma. The stromal elements show pleomorphism and atypia, though this is rarely of a striking degree, and contain more than 3, but less than 20, mitotic figures per 10 high power fields.

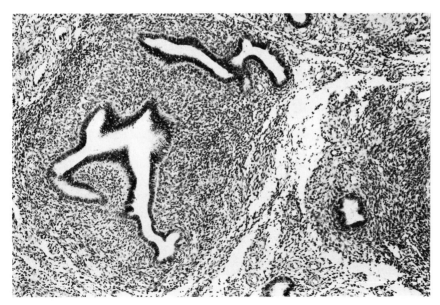

Figure 11.10   Müllerian adenosarcoma. Neoplastic glandular elements, lined by epithelium of endometrial type, are set in a cellular stroma. Haematoxylin and Eosin × 93.

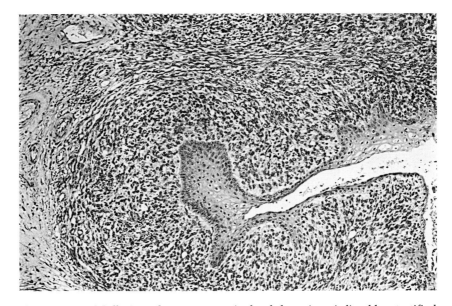

Figure 11.11 Müllerian adenosarcoma. A glandular acinus is lined by stratified squamous epithelium which exhibits a minor degree of cytological atypia. The stroma is highly cellular, mildly pleomorphic and contains a moderate number of mitoses. Haematoxylin and Eosin × 93.

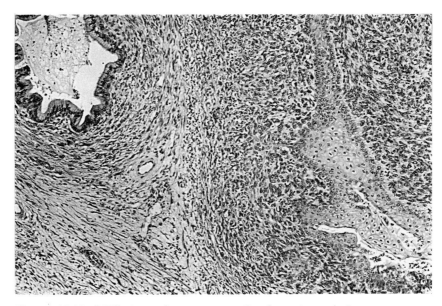

Figure 11.12 Müllerian adenosarcoma. Condensation of the sarcomatous stroma, forming a cambium layer, is particularly marked around the neoplastic gland to the right which is lined by stratified squamous epithelium. The gland to the left is lined by a single layer of mucus-secreting epithelium of cervical type, the cambium layer here is less striking. Haematoxylin and Eosin × 93.

Carcinofibromas, in which a malignant glandular component is supported by a prominent, but benign, stroma are extremely rare (Östör and Fortune, 1980; Thompson and Husemeyer, 1981). The epithelial component is usually an endometrioid adenocarcinoma whilst the stromal element resembles normal endometrial stroma; heterologous elements may be present (Chen and Vergon, 1981).

Carcinosarcomas appear to contain an intimate admixture of carcinomatous and sarcomatous elements, the relative proportions of which vary considerably (Sternberg *et al.*, 1954; Ober, 1959; Norris *et al.*, 1966; Norris and Taylor, 1966b; Chuang *et al.*, 1970; Kempson and Bari, 1970; Williamson and Christopherson, 1972; Barwick and LiVolsi, 1979; Fortune and Östör, 1987). Whether such neoplasms are genuinely carcinosarcomas or metaplastic (biphasic) carcinomas is currently a matter for debate.

Although sometimes anaplastic or very poorly differentiated (Figure 11.13), the carcinomatous component of a carcinosarcoma is often identical with an endometrioid type of endometrial adenocarcinoma (Figure 11.14) but can be, either in part or in whole, a tubal, endocervical or clear cell carcinoma. Bland, metaplastic squamous epithelium is not

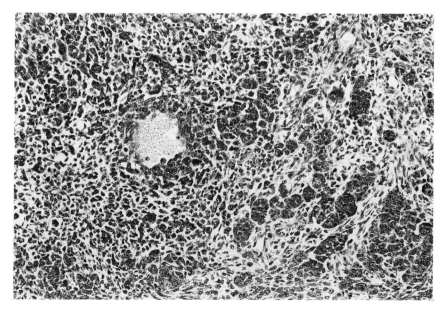

Figure 11.13 Carcinosarcoma. Poorly-defined and poorly-differentiated epithelial elements, to the right, are set in a sarcomatous stroma. It is difficult to distinguish the epithelial and sarcomatous components using morphological criteria alone. Haematoxylin and Eosin × 117.

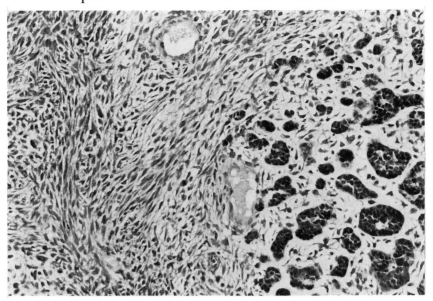

Figure 11.14 Carcinosarcoma. Well-defined glands lined by epithelium of uncertain type are seen on the right. The stroma in this area is largely undifferentiated. Haematoxylin and Eosin × 186.

uncommonly present within the acini of an endometrioid adenocarcinomatous element whilst occasionally there is a mixture of adenocarcinoma and squamous cell carcinoma; in rare instances the epithelial component is represented by a squamous cell carcinoma.

The non-epithelial component of a carcinosarcoma may resemble an endometrial stromal sarcoma (Figure 11.13) whilst, infrequently, a leiomyosarcomatous or fibrosarcomatous pattern predominates. Often, however, the appearances are those of a sarcoma of indeterminate type (Figure 11.14) and as Fortune and Östör (1987) have commented 'there is little point in agonising over the exact type of stroma present as this has no influence on prognosis'. The non-epithelial component is usually highly cellular, commonly lacks the 'cambium' layer formation which characterizes mixed Müllerian tumours of lesser malignancy and almost invariably shows conspicuous pleomorphism, atypia and mitotic activity. Bizarre tumour giant cells with grossly atypical nuclei are often present whilst mitotic figures number more than 20 per 10 high power fields and are frequently of markedly aberrant form. Small, rounded, eosinophilic, hyaline bodies of unknown nature have been noted in the stroma of mixed tumours of high grade malignancy and are, in our experience, a common and characteristic feature (Clement and Scully, 1988).

Heterologous components are present in about 50% of carcinosarcomas, malignant striated muscle, cartilage, bone and fat being the alien tissues most frequently encountered. The commonest heterologous component is striated muscle which is usually ,seen as scattered, occasionally aggregated, rhabdomyoblasts. These are typically 'strap' or 'tadpole' shaped and have cross striations which may be apparent in haematoxylin and eosin stained sections but are more easily identified in P.T.A.H. stained preparations (Figure 11.15). Relatively large, plump, rounded or 'racquet-shaped' cells with abundant fibrillary or granular cytoplasm and atypical nuclei are also often seen in mixed tumours of high grade malignancy (Figure 11.16) commonly in association with clearly definable rhabdomyoblasts but sometimes in the absence of such cells. The practice of classing such cells also as rhabdomyoblasts has been deplored by some who would maintain that cells only merit this categorization if they show either cross striations or electronmicroscopic evidence of skeletal muscle differentiation (Hendrickson and Kempson, 1980; Fortune and Östör, 1987). We do, however, regard these 'racquet' cells as rhabdomyoblasts and in defence of our apparently relaxed approach to diagnostic criteria would maintain that cells with visible cross

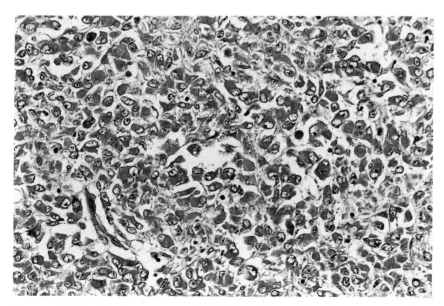

Figure 11.15 Carcinosarcoma. Rhabdomyoblasts in the stroma of a carcinosarcoma. The cells have copious eosinophilic cytoplasm and eccentric nuclei. It is rare to identify cross striations in such cells. Haematoxylin and Eosin × 297.

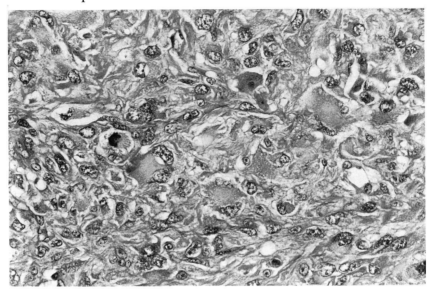

Figure 11.16 Carcinosarcoma. Within the stroma of the neoplasm there are large cells which have the features of rhabdomyoblasts. They have rather irregular outlines, eccentric nuclei and several are multinucleate. A mitosis is present just to the left of centre. Haematoxylin and Eosin × 370.

striations are immature rhabdomyocytes rather than rhabdomyoblasts. Immunocytochemical staining for myoglobulin might be expected to resolve any difficulties in identifying cells of striated muscle type (Mukai *et al.*, 1980) but in our hands this technique yields notably capricious results.

The second most common heterologous element in carcinosarcomas is cartilage which usually takes the form of chondrosarcomatous foci with large, atypical nuclei (Figure 11.17). Occasionally, however, the cartilaginous tissue is immature rather than overtly malignant (Figure 11.18). Osteosarcomatous elements are uncommon whilst any fat present in these tumours is usually due to degenerative changes rather than to heterologous liposarcoma.

11.4.2 *Differential diagnosis*

Both the adenofibroma and the adenosarcoma can be mistaken for a simple endometrial or endocervical polyp. Simple polyps do not, show papillary projections into clefts and cysts, lack any condensation of the stroma around the epithelial elements and differ from an adenosarcoma,

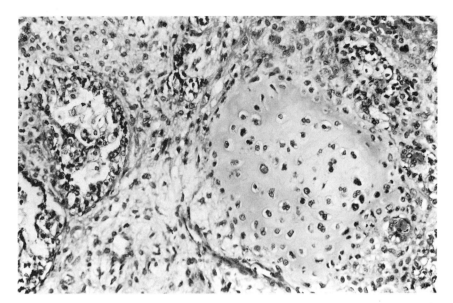

Figure 11.17 Carcinosarcoma with heterologous elements. The glands to the left are lined by clear cells similar to those seen in clear-celled carcinoma. The cartilaginous area, to the right, shows pleomorphism and the cells are hyperchromatic. Haematoxylin and Eosin × 186.

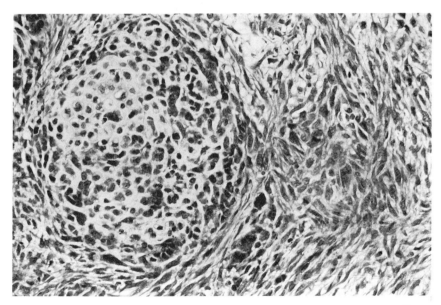

Figure 11.18 Carcinosarcoma. A focus of tissue resembling immature cartilage, to the left, is set in an undifferentiated sarcomatous stroma. Haematoxylin and Eosin × 232.

though not an adenofibroma, in having a bland stroma. Atypical polypoid adenomyomas (Chapter 8) also enter into the differential diagnosis of adenofibromas and adenosarcomas but are distinguished by the leiomyomatous nature of their stroma and their lack of a cambium layer. Differentiation of an adenosarcoma from a pure endometrial stromal sarcoma with entrapped normal endometrial glands is discussed on p. 201.

A carcinosarcoma has to be distinguished from a pure homologous or heterologous sarcoma and from an anaplastic carcinoma. The distinction from a pure sarcoma or carcinoma rests solely upon recognition of the biphasic pattern of a mixed tumour and this may not be possible in biopsy material which can contain tissue from only one component of such a neoplasm. Even if both epithelial and non-epithelial elements are present in curettage material they may be so intimately blended that their separate nature is not readily apparent. Under such circumstances staining for intermediate filaments would be expected to be of considerable value, the carcinomatous areas expressing keratins and epithelial membrane antigen (EMA) and the sarcomatous tissues desmin and/or vimentin. Unfortunately, whilst this staining pattern is usually found, the non-epithelial component may also stain positively for keratins and EMA whilst the epithelial tissue often also stains positively for vimentin (Bitterman et al., 1988). Benign heterologous elements may be seen very occasionally in the stroma of an endometrial adenocarcinoma (Nogales et al., 1982), but nevertheless the presence of such elements in what is clearly seen on biopsy as a malignant tumour should raise a strong suspicion of a mixed neoplasm as should the finding of bizarre cells with highly atypical nuclei.

Occasionally a carcinosarcoma which contains heterologous elements is confused with a teratoma; uterine teratomas are of extreme rarity (Chapter 12), occur usually in young patients rather than in elderly women and differ from mixed Müllerian tumours in their content of ectodermal and endodermal tissues.

In the very unusual circumstances of a carcinosarcoma occurring in childhood or in young women (Amr et al., 1986) it has to be distinguished from an embryonal rhabdomyosarcoma (sarcoma botyroides) arising in the cervix or vagina but being present in curetted material; the distinction again depends upon demonstration of a biphasic pattern in the mixed tumour and this can be impossible if the biopsy contains only heterologous rhabdomyosarcomatous tissue.

11.4.3   Assessment of malignancy in mixed tumours

The pathologist encountering a mixed tumour has to distinguish between the benign adenofibroma, the indolently malignant adenosarcoma and the highly aggressive carcinosarcoma. The distinction between an adenofibroma and an adenosarcoma can be difficult in biopsy material but cytological evidence of malignancy within the stromal component and the presence of heterologous elements point to a diagnosis of adenosarcoma. In doubtful cases, reliance has to be placed on the mitotic count in the neoplasm, tumours with less than 4 mitotic figures per 10 high power fields behaving as adenofibromas and those with 4 or more mitoses per 10 high power fields behaving, and being classified, as adenosarcomas (Mills *et al.*, 1981; Zaloudek and Norris, 1981b). The distinction between an adenosarcoma and a carcinosarcoma usually presents few difficulties; nevertheless occasional neoplasms fall into a grey hinterland between these two clearly defined entities and here it is necessary once again to resort to mitotic counts, neoplasms with 20 or more mitoses per 10 high power fields being regarded as of high grade malignancy.

It is doubtful if there are any histological features of carcinosarcomas of any prognostic significance. There is no convincing evidence that the presence or absence of heterologous elements is prognostically important, that the finding of cartilage in such neoplasms is a favourable feature or that tumours containing rhabdomyosarcomatous elements have an unusually gloomy prognosis (Fortune and Östör, 1987).

References

Amr, S.S., Tavassoli, F.A., Hassan, A.A., Issa, A.A. and Maddnat, F.A. (1986) Mixed mesodermal tumor of the uterus in a 4-year old girl. *Int. J. Gynecol. Pathol.*, **5**, 371–8.

Baggish, M.S. and Woodruff, J.D. (1972) Uterine stromatosis: clinicopathologic features and hormone dependency. *Obstet. Gynecol.*, **40**, 487–98.

Barwick, K.W. and LiVolsi, V.A. (1979) Malignant mixed Müllerian tumors of the uterus: a clinicopathologic assessment in 34 cases. *Am. J. Surg. Pathol.*, **3**, 125–35.

Bitterman, P., Chun, B.K. and Kurman, R.S. (1988) Uterine carcinosarcomas: a clinicopathologic and immunohistologic study providing evidence that these are biphasic carcinomas. *Mod. Pathol.*, **1**, 10a.

Bonazzi del Poggetto, C., Virtanen, I., Lehto, V-P, Wahlström, I. and Saksela, E. (1983) Expression of intermediate filaments in ovarian and uterine tumors. *Int. J. Gynecol. Pathol.*, **1**, 359–66.

Brown, D.C., Theaker, D.M., Banks, P.M., Gatter, K.C. and Mason, D.Y. (1987) Cytokeratin expression in smooth muscle tumours. *Histopathology*, **11**, 477–86.

Chen, K.T.K. (1985) Rhabdomyosarcomatous uterine adenosarcoma. *Int. J. Gynecol. Pathol.*, **4**, 146–52.

Chen, K.T.K. and Vergon, J.M. (1981) Carcinomesenchymoma of the uterus. *Am. J. Clin. Pathol.*, **75**, 746–8.

Chuang, J.T., Van Velden, D.J.J. and Graham, J.B. (1970) Carcinosarcomas and mixed mesodermal tumor of the uterine corpus: review of 49 cases. *Obstet. Gynecol.*, **35**, 769–80.

Clement, P.B. (1978) Chondrosarcoma of the uterus: report of a case and review of the literature. *Hum. Pathol.*, **9**, 726–32.

Clement, P.B. and Scully, R.E. (1974) Müllerian adenosarcoma of the uterus a clinicopathologic analysis of ten cases of a distinct type of Müllerian mixed tumor. *Cancer*, **34**, 1138–49.

Clement, P.B. and Scully, R.E. (1976) Uterine tumors resembling ovarian sex-cord tumors. *Am. J. Clin. Pathol.*, **69**, 276–83.

Clement, P.B. and Scully, R.E. (1988) Uterine tumors with mixed epithelial and mesenchymal elements. *Semin. Diagn. Pathol.*, **5**, 199–222.

Crum, C.P., Rogers, B.H. and Anderson, W. (1980) Osteosarcoma of the uterus: case report and review of the literature. *Gynecol. Oncol.*, **9**, 256–68.

Donkers, B., Kazzaz, B.A. and Meimering, H. (1972) Rhabdomyosarcoma of the corpus uteri: report of two cases with review of the literature. *Am. J. Obstet. Gynecol.*, **114**, 1025–30.

Ellis, P.S.J. and Whitehead, R. (1981) Mitosis counting: a need for reappraisal. *Hum. Pathol.*, **12**, 3–4.

Fekete, P.S. and Vellios, F. (1984) The clinical and histologic spectrum of endometrial stromal neoplasms: a report of 41 cases. *Int. J. Gynecol. Pathol.*, **3**, 198–212.

Fortune, D.W. and Östör, A.G. (1987) Mixed Müllerian tumours of the uterus. In *Haines and Taylor's Textbook of Obstetrical and Gynaecological Pathology* (ed. H. Fox), Churchill Livingstone, Edinburgh, pp. 457–77.

Fox, H., Harilal, K.R. and Youell, A. (1979) Müllerian adenosarcoma of the uterine body: a report of nine cases. *Histopathology*, **3**, 167–80.

Grimalt, M., Arghelles, M. and Ferenczy, A. (1975) Papillary cystadenofibroma of endometrium: a histochemical and ultrastructural study. *Cancer*, **36**, 137–44.

Hart, W.R. and Craig, J.R. (1978) Rhabdomyosarcoma of the uterus. *Am. J. Clin. Pathol.*, **70**, 217–23.

Hart, W.R. and Yoonessi, M. (1977) Endometrial stromatosis of the uterus. *Obstet. Gynecol.*, **49**, 393–403.

Hendrickson, M.R. and Kempson, R.L. (1980) *Surgical Pathology of the Uterine Corpus*, W.B. Saunders, Philadelphia.

Kempson, R.L. (1976) Mitosis counting. *Hum. Pathol.*, **7**, 482–3.

Kempson, R.L. and Bari, W. (1970) Uterine sarcomas: classification, diagnosis and prognosis. *Hum. Pathol.*, **1**, 331–49.

Kempson, R.L. and Hendrickson, M.R. (1987) Pure mesenchymal neoplasms of the uterine corpus. In *Haines and Taylor: Textbook of Obstetrical and Gynaecological Pathology* (ed. H. Fox), Churchill Livingstone, Edinburgh, pp. 411–56.

Marshall, R.J. and Braye, S.G. (1985) α-1-antitrypsin, α-1-antichymotrypsin, actin, and myosin in uterine sarcomas. *Int. J. Gynecol. Pathol.*, **4**, 346–54.

Martinelli, G., Pileri, S., Bazzochi, F. and Serra, L. (1980) Müllerian adenosarcoma of the uterus: a report of 5 cases. *Tumori*, **66**, 499–506.

Mills, S.E., Sugg, K.N. and Mahnesmith, R.C. (1981) Endometrial adenosarcoma with pelvic involvement following uterine perforation. *Diag. Gynecol. Obstet.*, **3**, 149–54.

Mukai, K., Varela-Duran, J. and Nochomouitz, L.F. (1980) The rhabdomyoblast in mixed Müllerian tumors of the uterus and ovary: an immunohistochemical study of myoglobin in 25 cases. *Am. J. Clin. Pathol.*, **74**, 101–4.

Nogales, F.F., Gomez-Morales, M., Raymundo, C. and Aguilar, D. (1982) Benign heterologous tissue components associated with endometrial carcinoma. *Int. J. Gynecol. Pathol.*, **1**, 286–91.

Norris, H.J. (1976) Mitosis counting. *Hum. Pathol.*, **7**, 483–4.

Norris, H.J. and Taylor, H.B. (1966a) Mesenchymal tumors of the uterus. I. A clinical and pathological study of 53 endometrial stromal tumors. *Cancer*, **19**, 755–66.

Norris, H.J. and Taylor, H.B. (1966b) Mesenchymal tumors of the uterus. III. A clinical and pathological study of thirty-one cases of carcinosarcoma. *Cancer*, **19**, 1459–65.

Norris, H.J., Roth, E. and Taylor, H.B. (1966) Mesenchymal tumors of the uterus. II. A clinical and pathological study of thirty-one mixed mesodermal tumors. *Obstet. Gynecol.*, **28**, 57–63.

Norton, A.J., Thomas, J.A. and Isaacson, P.G. (1987) Cytokeratin-specific monoclonal antibodies are reactive with tumours of smooth muscle derivation: an immunocytochemical and biochemical study using antibodies to intermediate filament cytoskeletal proteins. *Histopathology*, **11**, 487–96.

Ober, W.B. (1959) Uterine sarcomas: histogenesis and taxonomy. *Ann. N.Y. Acad. Sci.*, **75**, 568–85.

Östör, A.G. and Fortune, D.W. (1980) Benign and low grade variants of mixed Müllerian tumours of the uterus. *Histopathology*, **4**, 369–82.

Park, W.W. (1980) *The Histology of Borderline Cancer*, Springer-Verlag, Berlin.

Scully, R.E. (1976) Mitosis counting. *Hum. Pathol.*, **7**, 481–2.

Siegal, G.P., Taylor, L.L., Nelson, K.G., Reddick, R.L., Frazelle, M.M., Siegried, J.M., Walton, L.A. and Kaufman, D.G. (1983) Characterisation of a pure heterologous sarcoma of the uterus: rhabdomyosarcoma of the corpus. *Int. J. Gynecol. Pathol.*, **2**, 303–15.

Silverberg, S.G. (1976) Reproducibility of the mitosis count in the histologic diagnosis of smooth muscle tumors of the uterus. *Hum. Pathol.*, **7**, 451–4.

Sternberg, W.R., Clark, W.H. and Smith, R.C. (1954) Malignant mixed Müllerian tumor (mixed mesodermal tumor of the uterus): a study of twenty-one cases. *Cancer*, **7**, 704–24.

Tavassoli, F.A. and Norris, H.J. (1981) Mesenchymal tumors of the uterus. VII. A clinico-pathological study of 60 endometrial stromal nodules. *Histopathology*, **5**, 1–10.

Thompson, M. and Husemeyer, R. (1981) Carcinofibroma – a variant of the mixed Müllerian tumour: a case report. *Br. J. Obstet. Gynaecol.*, **88**, 1151–5.

Vakiani, M., Mawad, J. and Talerman, A. (1982) Heterologous sarcomas of the uterus. *Int. J. Gynecol. Pathol.*, **1**, 211–19.

Vellios, F., Ng, A.B.P. and Reagan, J.W. (1973) Papillary adenofibroma of the uterus: a benign mesodermal mixed tumor of Müllerian origin. *Am. J. Clin. Pathol.*, **60**, 543–51.

Williamson, E.O. and Christopherson, W.M. (1972) Malignant mixed Müllerian tumors of the uterus. *Cancer*, **29**, 585–92.

Yoonessi, M. and Hart, W.R. (1977) Endometrial stromal sarcomas. *Cancer*, **40**, 898–906.

Zaloudek, C.J. and Norris, H.J. (1981a) Mesenchymal tumors of the uterus. In *Progress in Surgical Pathology* III (eds C.M. Fenoglio and M. Wolff), Masson, New York, pp. 1–35.

Zaloudek, C.J. and Norris, H.J. (1981b) Adenofibroma and adenosarcoma of the uterus: a clinicopathologic study of 35 cases. *Cancer*, **48**, 354–66.

12 Non-Müllerian endometrial neoplasms

All the neoplasms described in this chapter are rare or, at best, uncommon in a uterine site. However, any may be encountered in curettings and all can give rise to considerable diagnostic confusion, especially if the pathologist is unaware that these tumours can occur in the uterus.

12.1 Vascular tumours

12.1 Haemangiopericytoma (Figure 12.1)

Uterine haemangiopericytomas can develop at any age. A proportion form polypoid masses within the uterine cavity and tissue from these tumours, which often cause complaints of abnormal vaginal bleeding, may thus appear in curettings (Greene and Gerbie, 1954; Silverberg *et al*, 1971; Sooriyaarachchi *et al.*, 1978; Buscema *et al.*, 1987).

The typical histological picture is of multiple vascular channels set amidst, and surrounded by, tightly-packed cells which may be arranged in trabeculae, nests or sheets. Characteristically the tumour cells in some areas are disposed concentrically around the vascular channels in an 'onion-skin' pattern. The tumour cells are rounded, polygonal or spindle shaped and have round or ovoid nuclei, a moderate amount of cytoplasm and ill-defined margins. The vascular channels range in size from small vessels of capillary calibre to wide sinusoids and form a ramifying network within the neoplasm. Very typically the dividing sinusoidal channels tend to have a 'stag horn' appearance. The vessels are lined by a single layer of endothelial cells which is often markedly attenuated. A reticulin stain shows that the vessels within the neoplasm are supported by a well-defined basal lamina and that reticulin fibres enmesh individual tumour cells to give a 'basket weave' appearance.

About 25% of uterine haemangiopericytomas behave in a malignant fashion but attempts to define those with a poor prognosis, in terms of

220

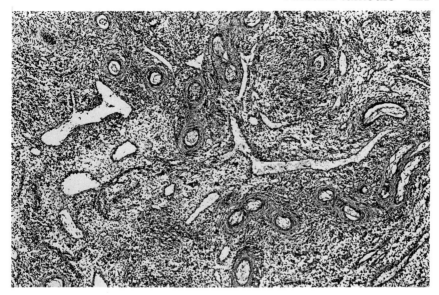

Figure 12.1   Haemangiopericytoma. The neoplasm has a cellular stroma in which can be identified the thin-walled, branching 'stag-horn' vessels as well as thick-walled vessels. Haematoxylin and Eosin × 60.

the degree of cytological atypia and pleomorphism, the presence of foci of necrosis and the number of mitotic figures, have not proved successful for haemangiopericytomas at this site (Buscema *et al.*, 1987).

Uterine haemangiopericytomas resemble closely the 'pericytic' type of endometrial stromal sarcoma of low grade malignancy, to the extent that many have maintained that all apparent uterine haemangiopericytomas are in fact misdiagnosed endometrial stromal sarcomas (Kempson and Hendrickson, 1987). We accept, however, uterine haemangio-pericytomas as a distinct entity and maintain that they can be recognized, even in curettings, by their content of irregular sinusoidal vessels, particularly those showing a branching 'stag horn' pattern. The fact that stromal sarcomas stain positively for alpha-1-antitrypsin and alpha-1-antichymotrypsin (Chapter 11) may be of some value in discriminating between the two neoplasms though it has to be admitted that, currently, information about the immunochemistry of haemangiopericytomas is scanty.

In some cases a distinction cannot be drawn in biopsy material between a haemangiopericytoma and a low grade endometrial sarcoma but, as both tumours necessitate a hysterectomy, this diagnostic impasse is of no great practical importance.

12.1.2 *Angiosarcoma*

Uterine angiosarcomas are rare but aggressive neoplasms (Ongkasuwan *et al.*, 1982; Witkin *et al.*, 1987). When encountered in curettings they may appear either as highly vascular neoplasms (Figure 12.2) or as undifferentiated tumours. If the tumour contains distinct vessels of irregular size and shape which communicate with each other to create an anastomosing vascular network the diagnostic problem becomes that of distinguishing an angiosarcoma from a haemangiopericytoma, endometrial stromal sarcoma or a highly vascular leiomyosarcoma. If the neoplasm is very poorly differentiated a quite different diagnostic problem is presented, namely its differentiation from a carcinoma, sarcoma or metastatic malignant melanoma. Recognition of a uterine angiosarcoma depends to a considerable extent upon an awareness that such neoplasms can occur at this site and most doubts as to the nature of the neoplasm can be removed in some, but unfortunately not all, cases by showing positive staining of the tumour cells with either factor VIII or *Ulex europica*, it being preferable to use both stains.

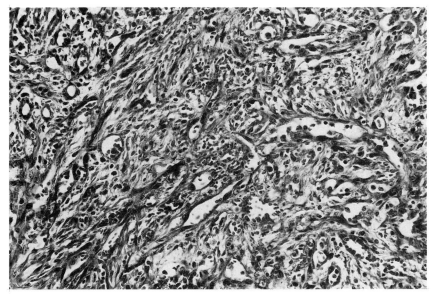

Figure 12.2   Angiosarcoma. The tumour consists of irregular, poorly-developed, thin-walled vascular channels lined by large cells. Haematoxylin and Eosin × 232.

12.2   Neural tumours

Both primitive neuroectodermal (Hendrickson and Scheithauer, 1986) and gliomatous neoplasms (Young *et al.*, 1981) of the endometrium may occur, their histogenesis being, to say the least, debatable. The primitive neuroectodermal tumours tend to show a predominantly neuro-blastomatous or medulloblastomatous pattern with focal glial or neuronal differentiation whilst the only reported gliomatous uterine tumour resembled a low grade fibrillary astrocytoma (Figure 12.3). Staining for glial fibrillary acidic protein has been generally positive in these exceedingly rare neoplasms.

Neoplastic glial tissue in an endometrial biopsy has to be differentiated from glial tissue which is present in the uterus as a fetal remnant. Fetal glial tissue not uncommonly evokes a mild, local chronic inflammatory

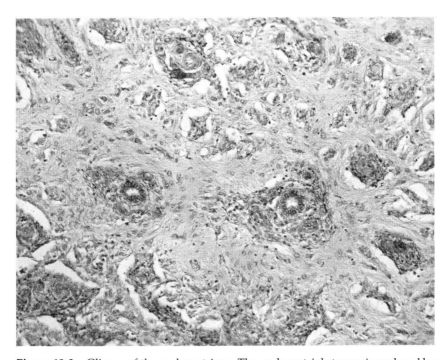

Figure 12.3   Glioma of the endometrium. The endometrial stroma is replaced by glial tissue which envelops inactive endometrial glands. The specimen is from the uterus of a 15 year old who presented with menorrhagia. Glial tissue formed a uterine mass and extensively infiltrated the myometrium. In these respects it differs from endometrial gliomatosis which it resembles histologically (Figure 8.11). (Photograph kindly supplied by Dr R.H. Young, Boston.)

cell infiltrate and is often admixed with other fetal tissues, such as cartilage or bone, whilst a history of recent abortion, the presence of chorionic villi or decidual tissue and the bland nature of the glial tissue will all point to a diagnosis of fetal remnants. Immature neural tissue may, however, be simply one component of a uterine teratoma or, most exceptionally, can occur as a heterologous element in a mixed Müllerian tumour of high grade malignancy. The finding in a biopsy of other mature tissue elements or of sarcomatous tissue will clearly be of value in establishing a correct diagnosis. Neural tumours, uterine teratomas containing immature neural elements and mixed Müllerian tumours are all indications for hysterectomy and the pathologist should not therefore suffer severe anxiety about difficulties encountered in differentiating these conditions. Fetal remnants do not, however, necessitate hysterectomy and every effort has to be made to draw a distinction between a primary neural neoplasm and these residues of a previous pregnancy.

Paraganglioma can also occur, albeit with extreme rarity, in the endometrium (Young and Thrasher, 1982). The appearances in a biopsy

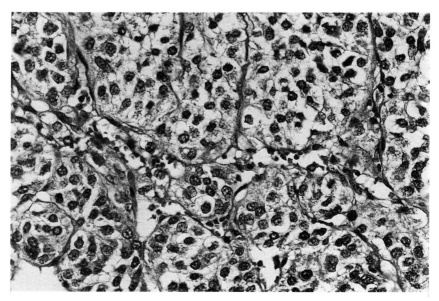

Figure 12.4 Non-chromaffin paraganglioma of the endometrium. The tumour forms the typical, clearly-defined nests of polygonal or round cells with clear or rather granular cytoplasm and round to oval nuclei. Haematoxylin and Eosin × 370.

specimen are characteristic of such neoplasms with tumour cells, containing abundant mildly eosinophilic cytoplasm and uniform vesicular nuclei, being arranged in nests which are limited by delicate fibrous septa containing prominent capillaries. In the only uterine paraganglioma which we have encountered (Figure 12.4) the principal diagnostic difficulty was in distinguishing it from an epithelioid leiomyoma growing into the uterine cavity. As with many of the rare neoplasms discussed in this chapter the diagnosis is very dependent upon the pathologist being aware that tumours of this type can occur in the uterus. The definitive diagnosis of uterine paragangliomas may rest upon electron microscopic identification of their content of typical granules, this being one of the few instances in which electron microscopy of an endometrial biopsy is of value.

Endometrial tumours having the general characteristic of para-gangliomas, but containing melanin granules, have also been described (Tavassoli, 1986); the true nature of these melanotic paragangliomas is uncertain.

12.3   Tumours of fat

Most, if not all, tumours reported as uterine lipomas have been, in reality, lipoleiomyomas with an unusually prominent lipomatous component (Dharkar et al., 1981; Pounder, 1982; Krenning and De Goey, 1983). The majority of such neoplasms are purely intramyometrial but in occasional cases the tumour protrudes into the uterine cavity and may thus be present in curettings. If, in a biopsy, mature fatty tissue is admixed with smooth muscle fibres the diagnosis of a lipoleiomyoma will be fairly clear but if purely fatty tissue is obtained the pathologist must consider the possibility that the fat is of fetal origin or is a component of a uterine teratoma. A history of recent pregnancy, histological evidence of a gestation and the presence of other fetal tissues will all indicate a diagnosis of fetal remnants whilst fatty tissue from a teratoma will usually be admixed with other mature elements. Perhaps the most important point the pathologist encountering fat in curettings should bear in mind is the possibility that the curette has perforated the uterus and has obtained omental tissue.

12.4   Miscellaneous soft tissue tumours

Malignant fibrous histiocytomas (Chou et al., 1985; Fujii et al., 1987), giant cell tumours (Kindblom and Seidal, 1981) and alveolar soft part sarcomas (Gray et al., 1986) have all been reported to occur in the uterus, with varying degrees of credibility. Biopsied tissue from such rare neoplasms may show diagnostically suggestive features, such as a storiform pattern, an alveolar arrangement of cells or the presence of osteoclast-like giant cells, but is more likely to appear simply as a poorly-differentiated sarcoma.

12.5   Germ cell and embryonic tumours

There have been a number of reasonably convincing reports of uterine teratomas (Martin *et al.*, 1979), usually of the mature cystic variety. Tissue in a biopsy from such a neoplasm has to be distinguished from fetal remnants, from cartilaginous or osseous metaplasia of the endometrial stroma and from a mixed Müllerian neoplasm with heterologous components. Most uterine teratomas have been detected in women of reproductive age and hence the most difficult to eliminate of these diagnostic alternatives is that of fetal remnants; the lack of a history of pregnancy, the absence of placental villi, decidua or hypersecretory endometrium together with the maturity of the teratomatous tissues and their haphazard relationship to each other will all suggest a teratoma rather than fetal remnants. Metaplastic cartilage or bone in the endometrial stroma can usually be seen to merge with stromal cells whilst the absence of endometrial stromal sarcomatous tissue and of either benign or malignant Müllerian type glands will eliminate the possibility of a mixed Müllerian neoplasm with heterologous elements.

Yolk sac tumours do occur in the endometrium though less commonly than in the vagina. They develop usually in children and can only be diagnosed in curettings if typical Schiller-Duval bodies are present.

A Wilm's tumour (Bittencourt *et al.*, 1981) and a retinal anlage tumour (Schultz, 1957) of the uterus have been described; both neoplasms occurred in children and both showed the typical appearances of such tumours as seen when encountered in more conventional sites.

12.6   Brenner tumour

A single, quite definite example of a uterine Brenner tumour has been reported (Arhelger and Bogian, 1976). Any pathologist unfortunate enough to encounter a further example of a neoplasm of this type in a biopsy would have to take into account the cytological blandness of the neoplastic cells when attempting to distinguish the tumour from a metastasis from a transitional cell carcinoma of the bladder or malignant Brenner tumour of the ovary.

12.7   Adenomatoid tumour

The vast majority of uterine adenomatoid tumours, now generally accepted as being of mesothelial origin, lie within the myometrium but, very exceptionally, tissue from such a neoplasm can be found in curettings (Carlier *et al.*, 1986). In a biopsy, an adenomatoid tumour may appear as an infiltrating neoplasm and the presence of signet ring cells may well rouse a suspicion of metastatic adenocarcinoma. Adenomatoid tumours give positive reactions with Alcian blue and Hale's colloidal iron, this reactivity being abolished by hyaluronidase. The adenomatoid tumours generally stain positively for keratin but there have been conflicting reports concerning their staining reactions for CEA and Factor VIII.

12.8   Lymphoma and leukaemia

Infiltration of the endometrium by lymphomatous or leukaemic cells (Figure 12.5) is not uncommon in women suffering from the advanced

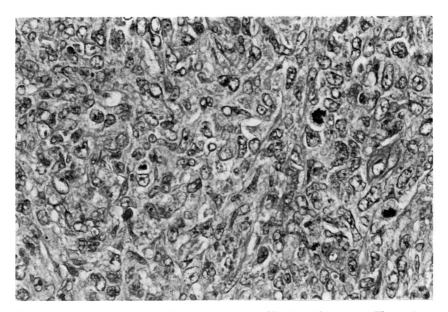

Figure 12.5 A non-Hodgkin's lymphomatous infiltrate in the uterus. The patient was a woman of 58 years in whom severe menorrhagia necessitated hysterectomy. The uterus, Fallopian tubes and one ovary were found to be heavily infiltrated by neoplastic cells. Haematoxylin and Eosin × 594.

stages of these diseases. On rare occasions, however, lymphomas present initially as an endometrial lesion, some of these having been confined to, and apparently arisen primarily at, this site (Fox and More, 1965; Harris and Scully, 1984; Chorlton, 1987). Lymphomas presenting as an endometrial lesion are usually of the non-Hodgkin's type though one instance of endometrial Hodgkin's disease has been noted (Hung and Kurtz, 1985). Granulocytic sarcoma may also occur in the endometrium (Kapadia *et al.*, 1978) whilst, very exceptionally, an endometrial lesion is the presenting feature of a chronic lymphatic leukaemia (Lucia *et al.*, 1952).

Endometrial lymphomas usually present as polypoid masses which cause abnormal vaginal bleeding and from which tissue is readily obtained by curettage. The characteristic histological appearance is that of a morphologically malignant, rather monotonous infiltrate, usually diffuse but sometimes with a nodular pattern. Infrequently the lymphomatous cells form cords and show an 'Indian file' pattern. Very typically, a lymphomatous infiltrate respects the normal endometrial structures, surrounding and infiltrating between, but not destroying, normal endometrial glands.

Recognition of lymphomatous or leukaemic infiltration of the endometrium depends primarily upon a degree of awareness of such a possibility by the pathologist and the differential diagnosis includes a dense inflammatory infiltrate, a 'lymphoma-like lesion', stromal cell sarcoma, poorly-differentiated carcinoma and metastatic carcinoma from an extragenital site. Carcinomas and sarcomas can often be distinguished from a lymphoma both in terms of their cytological features and their destructive, rather than infiltrative, growth pattern but the distinction from a metastatic lobular carcinoma of the breast can be exceptionally difficult. Stains for mucin, may, however, help to resolve this diagnostic dilemma. Staining for vimentin, desmin, epithelial membrane antigen and common leucocyte antigen will usually resolve any diagnostic doubts about distinguishing a lymphoma from an epithelial or mesenchymal neoplasm but still leaves the pathologist with the problem of differentiating a lymphoma from a severe chronic endometritis and from a 'lymphoma-like lesion'. In most cases of endometritis with an unusually dense chronic inflammatory cell infiltrate there is often destruction of the glandular tissue whilst the inflammatory nature of the infiltrate is usually revealed by the presence of ill-formed germinal centres, by the presence of tangible body macrophages and by the recognition that the inflammatory cells show a polymorphic, rather than a monomorphic, pattern. Whether or not a severe endometritis differs fundamentally from the 'lymphoma-like lesions' described by Young *et al.* (1985) is perhaps a moot point but these reactive lymphoid lesions of the endometrium have a typical appearance characterized by a heterogeneous pattern of large lymphoid cells of various types admixed with plasma cells, mature lymphocytes, neutrophil polymorphonuclear cells and eosinophils. The large lymphoid cells contain numerous mitotic figures and although usually forming ill-defined focal aggregates may be diffusely distributed. The histological pattern of a lymphoma-like lesion does therefore differ significantly from that of a genuine lymphoma and this is fortunate for Young *et al.* (1985) found that immunoperoxidase stains were of little value in distinguishing between benign and malignant lymphoid infiltration of the endometrium.

12.9 Metastatic tumour

Uterine metastases from extra-genital tumours are uncommon but pose a diagnostic trap for the unwary (Kaier and Holm-Jensen, 1972; Kumar and Hart, 1982; Kumar and Schneider, 1983; Bauer *et al.* 1984). Although a majority of such metastases are confined to the myometrium approximately one third involve the endometrium and will thus be apparent in endometrial curettings. The usual clinical presentation of a uterine

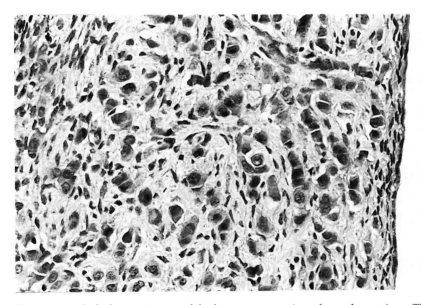

Figure 12.6 Lobular carcinoma of the breast metastatic to the endometrium. The neoplastic infiltrate is composed of small undifferentiated carcinoma cells with hyperchromatic nuclei and scanty cytoplasm arranged in Indian file. Haematoxylin and Eosin × 370.

metastasis is with abnormal vaginal bleeding or discharge and whilst there is a history of previous removal of an extragenital tumour in three quarters of the patients these symptoms represent the initial presentation of a primary extra-genital neoplasm in 25% of cases.

The primary tumours metastasizing most commonly to the uterus are, in descending order of frequency, carcinomas of the breast (particularly the lobular variety), colon, stomach and pancreas; less commonly metastases may arise from carcinomas of the kidney, bladder, gall bladder or thyroid whilst cutaneous malignant melanomas may also give rise to uterine metastases.

Commonly, metastatic tumours in endometrial curettings present a characteristic and diagnostic appearance with malignant cells infiltrating, singly, in cords or in clumps, normal endometrial stroma and surrounding normal endometrial glands. This appearance is seen particularly strikingly with metastatic lobular carcinoma of the breast (Figure 12.6), which characteristically retains its 'Indian-file' pattern, and

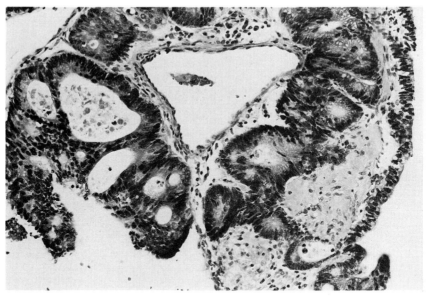

Figure 12.7 Colonic adenocarcinoma metastatic to the endometrium. The endometrium is infiltrated by a columnar cell, mucus-secreting adenocarcinoma. The patient, a woman of 64 years, was known to have had a rectal carcinoma resected nine months previously. She developed postmenopausal bleeding and curettage revealed fragments of carcinoma similar to that removed previously from the rectum. Haematoxylin and Eosin × 186.

with metastatic signet ring cell carcinomas of the stomach or colon. The differential diagnosis in such cases is from an endometrial stromal sarcoma, a Müllerian adenosarcoma, and a malignant lymphoma. Distinction from an endometrial stromal sarcoma rests upon noting the absence of a rich vascular background, the encompassing, rather than the destruction, of endometrial glands, the cytological characteristics of the infiltrating cells (which bear little or no resemblance to those of a stromal sarcoma) and, in many cases, the presence of mucin. Differentiation of a metastatic neoplasm from a Müllerian adenosarcoma is dependent, again, on the cytological features, the usually atrophic nature of the encircled endometrial glands, the absence of a cambium layer and the presence of mucin. In the occasional difficult case positive staining of the infiltrating cells for epithelial membrane antigens, keratins and, in the case of malignant melanoma, S-100 will usually resolve the diagnostic problem. The differential diagnosis from a lymphoma is discussed on p. 228.

Some metastases to the endometrium, however, may not show this typical infiltrative pattern and can present as a neoplastic mass which can be mistaken, in endometrial curettings, for a primary adenocarcinoma of the endometrium. This is particularly true for metastases from a colonic adenocarcinoma (Figure 12.7), which can mimic a primary mucinous carcinoma of the endometrium, and from renal adenocarcinoma, which can closely resemble a clear cell carcinoma of the endometrium.

References

Arhelger, R.E. and Bogian, J.J. (1976) Brenner tumor of the uterus. *Cancer*, **38**, 1741–3.

Bauer, R.D., McCoy, C.P., Roberts, D.K. and Fritz, G. (1984) Malignant melanoma metastatic to the endometrium. *Obstet. Gynecol.*, **63**, 264–7.

Bittencourt, A.L., Britto, J.F. and Fonseca, L.E. (1981) Wilm's tumor of the uterus: the first report in the literature. *Cancer*, **47**, 2496–9.

Buscema, J., Klein, V., Rotmensch, J., Rosenhein, N. and Woodruff, J.D. (1987) Uterine hemangiopericytoma. *Obstet. Gynecol.*, **69**, 104–8.

Carlier, M.T., Dardick, I., Lagace, A.F. and Steeram, V. (1986) Adenomatoid tumor of uterus: presentation in endometrial curettings. *Int. J. Gynecol. Pathol.*, 5, 69–74.

Chorlton, I. (1987) Malignant lymphoma of the female genital tract and ovaries. In *Haines and Taylor: Obstetrical and Gynaecological Pathology* (ed. H. Fox), Churchill Livingstone, Edinburgh, pp. 737–62.

Chou, S.T., Fortune, D., Beischer, N.A., McLeish, G., Castle, L.A., McKelvie, B.A. and Planner, R.S. (1985) Primary malignant fibrous histiocytoma of the uterus – ultrastructural and immunocytochemical studies of two cases. *Pathology*, **17**, 36–40.

Dharkar, D.D., Kraft, J.R. and Gangaoharem, D. (1981) Uterine lipomas. *Arch. Pathol. Lab. Med.*, **105**, 43–5.

Fox, H. and More, J.R.S. (1965) Primary malignant lymphoma of the uterus. *J. Clin. Pathol.*, **18**, 724–8.

Fujii, S., Kanzaki, H., Konishi, I., Yamabe, H., Okamura, H. and Mori, T. (1987) Malignant fibrous histiocytoma of the uterus. *Gynecol. Oncol.*, **26**, 319–30.

Gray, D.G., Glick, A.D., Kurtin, P.J. and Jones, H.W. (1986) Alveolar soft part sarcoma of the uterus. *Hum. Pathol.*, **17**, 297–300.

Greene, R.R. and Gerbie, A.B. (1954) Hemangiopericytoma of the uterus. *Obstet. Gynecol.*, **3**, 150–61.

Harris, N.L. and Scully, R.E. (1984) Malignant lymphoma and granulocytic sarcoma of the uterus and vagina: a clinicopathologic analysis of 27 cases. *Cancer*, **53**, 2530–45.

Hendrickson, M.R. and Scheithauer, B.W. (1986) Primitive neuroectodermal tumor of the endometrium: report of two cases, one with electron microscopic observations. *Int. J. Gynecol. Pathol.*, **5**, 249–59.

Hung, L.H. and Kurtz, D.M. (1985) Hodgkin's disease of the endometrium. *Arch. Pathol. Lab. Med.*, **109**, 762–4.

Kaier, W. and Holm-Jensen, S. (1972) Metastases to the uterus. *Acta Pathol. Microbiol. Scand.*, **80**, 835–40.

Kapadia, S.B., Krause, J.R., Kanbour, A.I. and Hartsock, R.J. (1978) Granulocytic sarcoma of the uterus. *Cancer*, **41**, 687–91.

Kempson, R.L. and Hendrickson, M.R. (1987) Pure mesenchymal tumours of the uterine corpus. In *Haines and Taylor: Obstetrical and Gynaecological Pathology* (ed. H. Fox), Churchill Livingstone, Edinburgh, pp. 411–56.

Kindblom, L.G. and Seidal, T. (1981) Malignant giant cell tumour of the uterus. *Acta Path. Microbiol. Scand. Sect. A.*, **89**, 179–84.

Krenning, R.A. and De Goey, W.B. (1983) Uterine lipomas: review of the literature. *Clin. Exp. Obstet. Gynecol.*, **10**, 91–4.

Kumar, A. and Schneider, V. (1983) Metastases to the uterus from extrapelvic primary tumors. *Int. J. Gynecol. Pathol.*, **2**, 134–40.

Kumar, N.B. and Hart, W.R. (1982) Metastases to the uterine corpus from extragenital cancers: a clinicopathologic study of 63 cases. *Cancer*, **50**, 2163–9.

Lucia, S.P., Mills, H., Lowenhaupt, E. and Hunt, M.L. (1952) Visceral involvement in primary neoplastic diseases of the reticuloendothelial system. *Cancer*, **5**, 1193–200.

Martin, E., Scholes, J., Richart, R.M. and Fenoglio, C.M. (1979) Benign cystic teratoma of the uterus. *Am. J. Obstet. Gynecol.*, **135**, 429–31.

Ongkasuwan, C., Taylor, J.E., Tang, C.K. and Prempree, T. (1982) Angiosarcomas of the uterus and ovary. *Cancer*, **49**, 1469–75.

Pounder, D.J. (1982) Fatty tumours of the uterus. *J. Clin. Pathol.*, **35**, 1380–3.

Schultz, D.M. (1957) A malignant melanotic neoplasm of the uterus, resembling the 'retinal anlage' tumor. *Am. J. Clin. Pathol.*, **28**, 524–33.

Silverberg, S.G., Wilson, M.A. and Board, J.A. (1971) Hemangiopericytoma of the uterus: an ultrastructural study. *Am. J. Obstet. Gynecol.*, **110**, 397–404.

Sooriyaarachchi, G.S., Ramirez, G. and Roley, E.L. (1978) Hemangiopericytoma of the uterus: report of a case with a comprehensive review of the literature. *J. Surg. Oncol.*, **10**, 399–408.

Tavassoli, F.A. (1986) Melanotic paraganglioma of the uterus. *Cancer*, **58**, 942–8.

Witkin, G.B., Askin, F.B., Geratz, J.D. and Reddick, R.L. (1987) Angiosarcoma of the uterus: a light microscopic, immunohistochemical and ultrastructural study. *Int. J. Gynecol. Pathol.*, **6**, 176–84.

Young, R.H., Harris, N.L. and Scully, R.E. (1985) Lymphoma-like lesions of the lower female genital tract: a report of 16 cases. *Int. J. Gynecol. Pathol.*, **4**, 289–99.

Young, R.H., Kleinman, G.M. and Scully, R.E. (1981) Glioma of the uterus: report of a case with comments on histogenesis. *Am. J. Surg. Pathol.*, **5**, 695–9.

Young, T.W. and Thrasher, T.V. (1982) Non-chromaffin paraganglioma of the uterus: a case report. *Arch. Pathol. Lab. Med.*, **106**, 608–9.

13 The endometrium in normal and abnormal pregnancy

A high proportion of curettings received in most pathology laboratories are from women who are, or have very recently been, pregnant and it is important therefore that the pathologist be conversant with the normal pattern of pregnancy-induced changes in the endometrium. A knowledge of the processes of implantation and placentation is also of value in interpreting those biopsies which include the implantation site (the 'placental site reaction').

It is recognized, of course, that the endometrium of a woman with a very early normal pregnancy is rarely deliberately sampled. Occasional biopsies will, however, be received from unsuspected early pregnancies, these, ironically, often having been taken for investigation of infertility. Usually, curettage during, or immediately after, pregnancy is, apart from therapeutic abortion, undertaken because the gestation has not followed a normal course, being ectopically situated, ending prematurely in abortion or being attended by post-partum complications.

In an increasing number of centres, post-partum placental bed biopsies will also be received. These are taken principally for an assessment of the adequacy and extent of conversion of spiral arteries into uteroplacental vessels and are of great value in the study of pregnancies complicated by pre-eclampsia or fetal intrauterine growth retardation. Biopsies of this type lie outside the remit of this text however, and those wishing to pursue further this important topic are referred to an excellent review (Robertson *et al.*, 1986).

13.1 Pregnancy-induced changes in the endometrium

If conception occurs during the course of a normal menstrual cycle the blastocyst will begin to implant in the endometrium at about the 9th post-ovulatory day, i.e. during the mid-secretory phase of the cycle. Secretion of hCG from the blastocyst prevents decay of the corpus luteum and thus progesterone levels fail to decline and progesterone-induced changes in the endometrium persist. Hence an endometrial biopsy taken during

234

days 25–28 of a cycle in which conception has occurred will show a well-marked predecidual change, together with considerable residual oedema, in the stroma, well-developed spiral arterioles and continuing secretory activity in the endometrial glands. If implantation is successful, unabated secretory activity will continue in the endometrial glands and within a few weeks a hypersecretory pattern will emerge (Figure 13.1) with the glandular epithelium becoming increasingly vacuolated and thrown into pseudopapillary folds. Towards the end of the first trimester this hypersecretory pattern will begin to regress and the glands subsequently become inactive and involuted. In many, but by no means all, cases a focal Arias-Stella change will be present within the endometrium of the gravid woman, this phenomenon usually not becoming apparent until after the 5th week of pregnancy. This is characterized by excessively convoluted glands, the epithelial cells of which have abundant clear cytoplasm, extensively vacuolated by glycogen, and nuclei showing variable degrees of pleomorphism, hyperchromasia and atypia (Figure 13.2). Irregular stratification and papillary tufting, or infolding, of the epithelial cells are characteristic features. An Arias-Stella change is thought to be due to the action of hCG on the endometrium and, as such, its presence in a biopsy simply

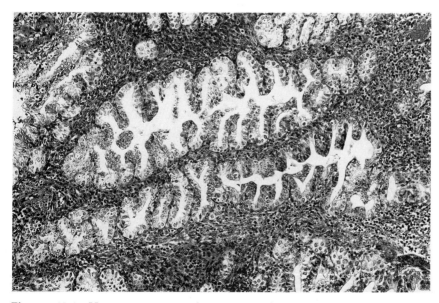

Figure 13.1 Hypersecretory endometrium of pregnancy. The glandular serrations are particularly prominent, almost forming papillae, and the glandular epithelium is secretory. Haematoxylin and Eosin × 117.

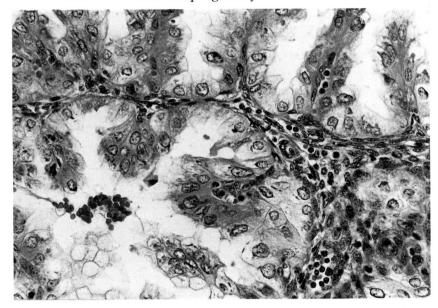

Figure 13.2 Arias-Stella change. The glandular epithelium exhibits hypersecretory features and the nuclei have lost their polarity. The epithelium forms small tufts which protrude into the glandular lumina. Note the absence of epithelial mitoses and the normal distribution of the nuclear chromatin. Haematoxylin and Eosin × 370.

indicates that trophoblastic tissue is present, either in an intrauterine or ectopic site and either as a component of a normal pregnancy or as part of a hydatidiform mole or choriocarcinoma. The focal nature of this hormonally-induced change is a curious, currently unexplained fact.

The predecidual stromal cells present towards the end of a cycle in which fertilization has occurred soon become converted into true decidual cells, increasing in size, having pale nuclei with prominent nucleoli, abundant cytoplasm and sharply defined borders. As the stromal oedema regresses these cells form solid sheets which are progressively infiltrated by K-cells, these being granulated lymphoid cells whose function is uncertain (Bulmer *et al.*, 1987).

13.2 Placentation and the development of the placental site reaction

Soon after implantation, probably between the 15th and 20th post-ovulatory days, the developing fetal placenta is separated from the decidua by the trophoblastic shell into which anchoring villi are inserted via their distal cytotrophoblastic cell columns. Extravillous cytotropho-blastic cells from the tips of the anchoring villi penetrate the trophoblastic shell and stream out to colonize the decidua and adjacent myometrium of the placental bed, these cells forming the interstitial extravillous cyto-trophoblastic cell population (also sometimes referred to as 'intermediate trophoblastic cells'). The extent of the invasion of the placental bed by cytotrophoblastic cells has been seriously underestimated in the past and many of the cells which at first sight appear to be decidual are in fact trophoblastic (Pijnenborg et al., 1980). As pregnancy progresses many of the infiltrating interstitial cytotrophoblastic cells regress whilst those remaining tend increasingly to fuse and form multinucleated syncytio-trophoblastic-like cells which are particularly aggregated at the junction of the endometrium and myometrium.

Extravillous cytotrophoblastic cells also stream into the lumens of the intradecidual portions of the spiral arteries of the placental bed where they often form intraluminal cellular plugs. These intravascular cytotrophoblastic cells destroy and replace the endothelial cells of the invaded vessels and then infiltrate the media with resulting destruction of the medial elastic and muscular tissue (Brosens et al., 1967); the arterial wall becomes replaced by fibrinoid material which is derived partly from fibrinogen in the maternal blood and partly from proteins secreted by the trophoblastic cells. At a later stage of gestation, between the 14th and 16th week, there is a resurgence of intravascular trophoblastic migration, with a second wave of cells moving down into the intramyometrial segments of the spiral arteries. Within the intramyometrial portion of these vessels the same process as occurs in their intradecidual portion is repeated, i.e. replacement of the endothelium, invasion and destruction of the medial musculo-elastic tissue and fibrinoid change in the vessel wall. The end result of this trophoblastic invasion and attack upon the vessels of the placental bed is that the thick-walled muscular spiral arteries are converted into flaccid, sac-like uteroplacental vessels which can passively dilate in order to accommodate the greatly augmented blood flow through this vascular system which is required as pregnancy progresses.

The practical aspect of this process of trophoblastic invasion of the placental bed and its contained vessels is the 'placental site reaction' which is often seen in biopsies from gravid uteri. In biopsies from first trimester pregnancies the placental site reaction will be apparent as mononuclear and multinucleated trophoblastic cells infiltrating the decidua (Figure 13.3) with trophoblastic cells within intradecidual spiral arteries (Figure 13.4) both in their lumens and in their walls, the invaded vessels showing fibrinoid necrosis. In biopsies from term pregnancies the placental site reaction is apparent mainly as multinucleated syncytiotrophoblastic-like cells within the placental bed; no trophoblastic

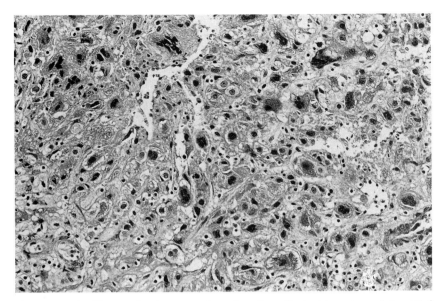

Figure 13.3 Placental site reaction in the first trimester. Interstitial cytotrophoblast cells are seen infiltrating the decidua. Some of the cells have become converted to syncytial placental bed giant cells. Haematoxylin and Eosin × 186.

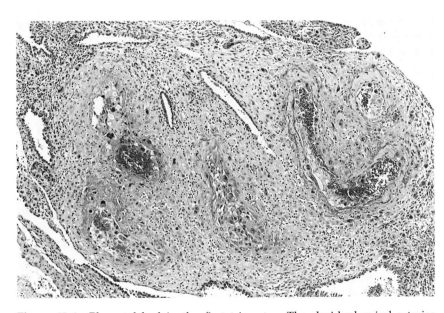

Figure 13.4 Placental bed in the first trimester. The decidual spiral arteries contain cytotrophoblast both in their lumens and in their walls. The vessels are dilated and fibrinoid material has been laid down in the walls. Haematoxylin and Eosin × 75.

cells will be apparent at this stage in the widely-dilated uteroplacental vessels.

The trophoblastic site reaction may be difficult in some cases to identify for the invading trophoblastic cells may closely resemble those of the decidua. The trophoblastic cells do, however, differ from decidual cells in giving a somewhat erratic positive staining reaction for human placental lactogen (hPL) and a consistently positive reaction for cytokeratins.

Four points require stressing. Firstly, the placental site reaction is the morphological hallmark of successful placentation. It is a physiological process and the term 'syncytial endometritis', which is sometimes applied to the placental site reaction, is totally inappropriate. Secondly, a placental site reaction is the only absolute indicator of an intrauterine pregnancy for placental villi and fetal tissue within the uterus could be derived from an intrauterine abortion of a tubal pregnancy. Thirdly, the degree of prominence of the placental site reaction at term varies considerably. A very marked placental site reaction can be confused with a placental site trophoblastic tumour or even with a choriocarcinoma; the differentation of these conditions is discussed in Chapter 14. Fourthly, the process of placentation results, for reasons which are far from clear, in focal necrosis of the decidua of the placental bed. This change is not seen in the decidua capsularis or in the decidua vera away from the placental bed. The necrotic areas are infiltrated by polymorphonuclear leucocytes and this change should be recognized in the placental bed as a physiological phenomenon and not classed as a 'deciduitis'.

13.3   Endometrial biopsy in ectopic pregnancy

Endometrial biopsies are often received from women with an ectopic pregnancy, curettage usually being performed for what is erroneously thought to be an incomplete abortion of an intrauterine gestation. Less commonly the endometrium is biopsied as part of the investigation of a woman with pelvic pain or an adnexal mass whilst, rather rarely, confirmation is sought that the endometrial morphology is in accord with a clinical diagnosis of ectopic pregnancy.

The appearances of the endometrium from a woman with an ectopic pregnancy will depend upon whether the fetus or embryo is alive or dead and, if dead, the time interval that has elapsed between fetal demise and endometrial sampling. An ectopic pregnancy is, in all respects other than the site of nidation, a normal gestation (Randall et al., 1987); hCG is produced by the ectopic trophoblast and there is a normally functioning corpus luteum of pregnancy. If the ectopically sited fetus is still alive at the time of biopsy the endometrium will show the changes characteristic of the pregnant state with decidualization of the stroma and

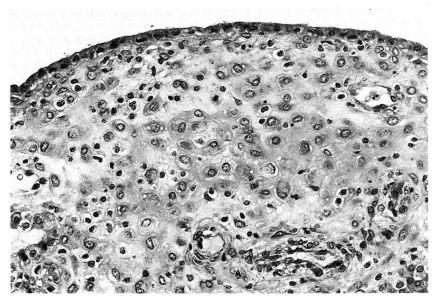

Figure 13.5 'Clean decidua' from a patient with an ectopic pregnancy. There is no placental site reaction in the uterus and the decidua, whilst exhibiting the features associated with pregnancy, is devoid of inflammation and necrosis. Spiral arteries in such cases become well-muscularized but show no evidence of transformation to uteroplacental vessels. Haematoxylin and Eosin × 297.

hypersecretory changes in the glands; a focal Arias-Stella change is present in 60–70% of cases (Bernhardt *et al.*, 1966) though, as already remarked, this change does not specifically indicate an extrauterine gestation. The endometrium from a woman with an ectopic pregnancy has a characteristically 'clean' appearance (Figure 13.5) without any of the decidual necrosis and inflammatory cell infiltration that characterizes an intrauterine gestation (Robertson, 1981). No placental villi, extraplacental fetal membranes or fetal tissues will be seen and, even more importantly, no evidence will be found of a placental site reaction; there will be a complete absence of any trophoblastic infiltration of the decidua, no trophoblastic invasion of the spiral arteries and no evident transformation of spiral arteries into uteroplacental vessels.

Following death of an ectopically-sited fetus the entire uterine lining may be sloughed off as a decidual cast, this showing the typically 'clean' appearance noted above. More commonly, the decidua disintegrates and is irregularly shed, a biopsy taken at this stage showing a crumbling decidua with areas of haemorrhage, necrosis and inflammation. Appearances similar to these are often found after abortion of an intrauterine pregnancy and hence it is under these circumstances that an assiduous search for placental villi or a placental site reaction is mandatory. If there has been a prolonged interval between fetal death and endometrial biopsy the decidua may have been completely shed and replaced by a proliferative endometrium which, because the first two cycles after an ectopic pregnancy tend to be anovulatory, may show a picture of a prolonged proliferative phase or an early simple hyperplasia (Robertson, 1981).

Many potential pitfalls await those studying endometrial biopsies from possible cases of ectopic pregnancy and it is wise to avoid dogmatic statements. The appearances of an endometrial biopsy may be compatible with, and indeed highly suggestive of, an ectopic pregnancy but are *never* diagnostic of an extrauterine gestation. The finding of 'clean' decidua lacking a placental site reaction, together with an absence of placental villi and fetal parts, is suggestive of an ectopic pregnancy but an identical appearance can, on occasion, be seen in biopsies following abortion of an intrauterine gestation, particularly if the biopsy contains only tissue from the decidua capsularis or the decidua basalis away from the placental site. Conversely, an intrauterine pregnancy should not be diagnosed solely on the basis of finding decidual tissue showing focal necrosis and inflammation. To sustain a diagnosis of an intrauterine pregnancy it is necessary to identify placental tissue, fetal parts or a placental site reaction within the curetted tissue. The purist would, pedantically but factually, maintain that in fact only a placental site reaction in an endometrial biopsy specimen is an absolute proof of an intrauterine gestation for, as already remarked, a tubal pregnancy may abort into the uterine cavity with subsequent retrieval of fetal or placental tissue on curettage.

A final, somewhat esoteric but real, possibility is that a woman may have concurrent intrauterine and ectopic pregnancies (Das, 1975; Honoré and Nickerson, 1977); hence, histological proof of an intrauterine pregnancy in a woman who is thought, on clinical grounds, to have an ectopic gestation does not completely negate the clinical diagnosis.

13.4   Endometrial biopsy in spontaneous abortion

Approximately 15% of established pregnancies spontaneously abort; curettage is commonly performed in such cases, usually because the abortion is thought to be incomplete with retention of 'products of conception'. Curettage under these circumstances is therefore primarily for therapeutic rather than diagnostic purposes but, nevertheless, the material obtained is usually submitted for pathological examination, partly for confirmation that an intrauterine pregnancy has actually been present and partly to exclude any possibility of gestational trophoblastic disease.

The material received from an abortion can range from a complete fetus and placenta to a few fragments of necrotic decidual tissue. If a fetus is present this should be submitted to a 'mini-autopsy', details of which have been fully provided elsewhere (Berry, 1980). In the majority of cases, however, a recognizable fetus is not macroscopically evident and the curetted material consists of a mixture of blood clot, partially necrotic decidual tissue, fragments of pregnancy-type endometrium and first trimester-type placental villi; under these circumstances there will be no difficulty in confirming that a gestation has been present. If placental villi are absent, a not uncommon event, a search should be made for a placental site reaction, identification of which provides unequivocal evidence of a recent intrauterine pregnancy. If neither placental villi nor a placental site reaction are detected the pathologist will be unable to confirm a recent uterine gestation, and should comment on the possibility of an ectopic pregnancy. The pathologist should *never* accept the presence of decidual tissue, unaccompanied by trophoblast, as confirmation of a pregnancy for the changes in the stroma evoked by exogenous progestagens can mimic closely those of true decidua.

The pathologist should also be very cautious of making a diagnosis of a 'septic abortion'. As already remarked, patchy decidual necrosis, with an inflammatory cell infiltrate, is a physiological phenomenon and the degree of inflammation in an abortion may be further increased as a response to tissue breakdown and the presence of a dead fetus. The possibility of a 'septic' abortion should therefore only be raised if there is a very marked inflammatory cell infiltrate, involving not only the decidua but also the hypersecretory glands and stroma of the endometrium well away from the placental site.

If trophoblastic tissue is present in curettage material received from an abortion it is usually easy to rule out the presence of trophoblastic disease (Chapter 14), especially if the importance of trophoblastic hyperplasia as a criterion for the diagnosis of a hydatidiform mole is borne in mind. Two difficulties sometimes arise. Firstly, the degree of trophoblastic proliferation in a normal first trimester placenta can be as great, or even greater, than that seen in a hydatidiform mole. In the normal placenta, however, the proliferation of trophoblast is always at one side or at one pole of a villus whilst in a mole it tends to be either multifocal or circumferential. The error of misinterpreting normal proliferating trophoblast as a choriocarcinoma is easily avoided if it is remembered that the presence of placental villi rules out a diagnosis of choriocarcinoma. Secondly, a hydropic abortion may be confused with a hydatidiform mole, particularly one of the partial variety. The term 'hydropic abortion'

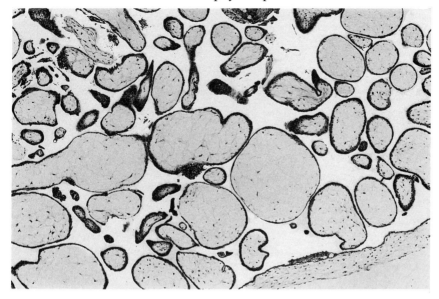

Figure 13.6 Hydropic abortus. The villi are swollen and hydropic. They are rounded and their trophoblastic mantle is attenuated. There are no fetal vessels. Haematoxylin and Eosin × 47.

is applied to the presence of swollen, oedematous, avascular villi which are rarely if ever sufficiently distended to be macroscopically visible; these villi are usually admixed with others of normal form and size but they can be distinguished from the vesicular villi of a partial hydatidiform mole by their smooth rounded contour and by their covering mantle of markedly attenuated trophoblast (Figure 13.6). These features contrast sharply with the strikingly irregular profile and the focal trophoblastic hyperplasia seen in the vesicular villi of a partial mole. A hydropic abortion is usually correctly equated with gross abnormality of the fetus and early fetal demise (the so-called 'blighted ovum') but occasional hydropic villi are sometimes encountered in placental tissue from recently dead fetuses and from therapeutic abortions.

Having confirmed the presence of a recent intrauterine gestation and having excluded trophoblastic disease the pathologist may well feel that no further information can be derived from examination of curettings from spontaneous abortions. Rushton (1987) has pointed out the value of commenting on the appearances of the placental villi in such curettings. In general terms the placental villi in abortion material may be hydropic, may be non-hydropic but show changes which have occurred as a consequence of fetal death, i.e. stromal fibrosis and sclerosis of the fetal

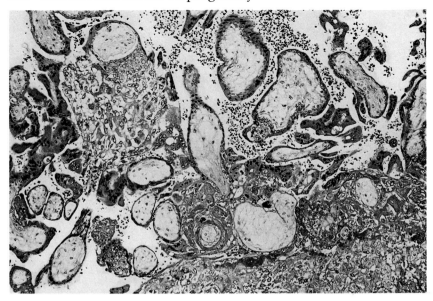

Figure 13.7 Spontaneous abortion. The stroma in many of the villi has undergone fibrosis secondary to fetal death. There is also sclerosis of many of the fetal vessels. Haematoxylin and Eosin × 93.

vessels (Figure 13.7), or be well vascularized and have a fully normal first trimester pattern (Figure 13.8). If there is widespread hydropic change, the distended villi being mixed with others of normal size but showing post-mortem changes, it is reasonable to assume that fetal demise has occurred at an early stage of pregnancy, the most probable cause of this being a gross fetal malformation or a fetal chromosomal abnormality. It is certainly clear that in a hydropic abortion the woman has aborted because the fetus has died. If, by contrast, the placental villi are well vascularized and show a normal first trimester pattern it is probable that the fetus has died because the patient has aborted, the most probable causes of an abortion of this type being in the fetal environment rather than intrinsic to the fetus, e.g. uterine malformations, immunological factors. If the placental villi show the postmortem changes of stromal fibrosis and obliteration of the fetal vessels it is again possible to deduce that abortion has occurred as a consequence of fetal death and that the factor leading to abortion is more likely to be intrinsic to the fetus than in its environment, though this is less certain than is the case with a hydropic abortus. The appearances of the placental villi give some indication therefore of the possible cause of an abortion and this, though of little importance in any

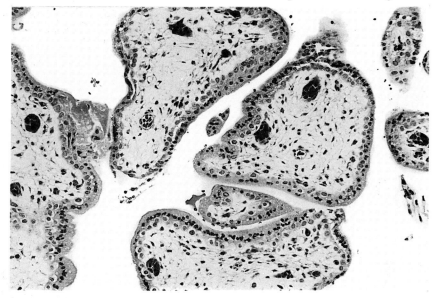

Figure 13.8 Normal first trimester placental villi. The villi contain a small number of fetal blood vessels in which red blood cells can be seen. Their stroma is immature and the covering trophoblast is composed of two clearly discernible layers, the inner cytotrophoblastic layer and the outer syncytial layer. Haematoxylin and Eosin × 186.

single abortion, can assume some significance in women who repeatedly abort.

Finally, the pathologist should examine the placental tissue in an abortion for evidence of a villitis. Maternal infections, such as toxoplasmosis, rubella or listeriosis, are a recognized cause of abortion and infections such as these can produce specific and diagnostic changes in the villi. Most cases of villitis are, however, of unknown aetiology. Those wishing for a full account of the histopathology of placental infections are referred to a recent review (Russell, 1987).

13.5 Postpartum bleeding

Postpartum bleeding is often thought to be commonly due to retention within the uterus of a portion of the placenta. Curettage in such cases occasionally reveals a mixture of blood clot and fibrotic placental villi (the so-called 'placental polyp') (Figure 13.9) but this is very much the exception rather than the rule. In some instances of postpartum bleeding there may be evidence of low grade uterine infection (Gibbs *et al.*, 1975)

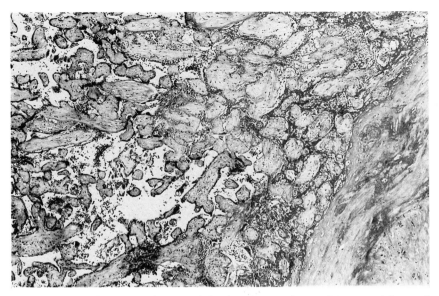

Figure 13.9 A fragment of retained third trimester placental tissue, a 'placental polyp' from a patient who complained of postpartum haemorrhage. Many of the villi are ghost-like and closely packed. Haematoxylin and Eosin × 60.

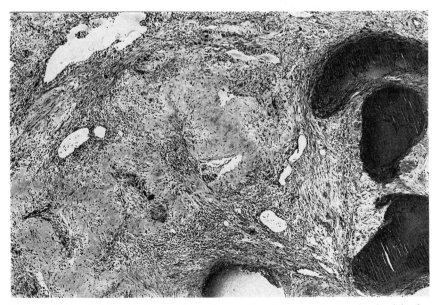

Figure 13.10 Subinvolution of the placental bed in a patient who had had a spontaneous abortion some weeks previously. The uteroplacental vessels to the left show changes of early involution, with recanalization of their thrombosed lumens. The vessels to the right remain widely patent and their lumens contain fresh blood clot. Haematoxylin and Eosin × 60.

but in the vast majority of cases postpartum bleeding appears to be due to inadequate or delayed involution of the placental bed (Robertson, 1981). The mechanism of uterine involution following pregnancy is ill understood but the major factors limiting blood loss from the placental site after delivery are spasm and thrombosis of the uteroplacental vessels; following thrombotic occlusion of these vessels, they collapse and undergo rapid involution. In cases of delayed involution curettage specimens contain hyalinized decidua, often with a population of 'ghost' trophoblastic cells, in which are set distended, partly hyalinized vessels that are incompletely occluded by thrombus (Figure 13.10). Very often both fresh and old thrombi are seen in the vessels and these appearances suggest that adequate thrombotic occlusion of the uteroplacental vessels was not attained at delivery, this leading to postpartum bleeding.

References

Bernhardt, R.N., Bruns, P.D. and Druse, V.E. (1966) Atypical endometrium associated with ectopic pregnancies. *Obstet. Gynecol.*, **28**, 849–53.

Berry, C.O. (1980) The examination of embryonic and fetal material in diagnostic histopathology laboratories. *J. Clin. Pathol.*, **38**, 317–26.

Brosens, I., Robertson, W.B. and Dixon, H.G. (1967) The physiological response of the vessels of the placental bed in normal pregnancy. *J. Pathol. Bacteriol.*, **93**, 569–79.

Bulmer, J.N., Hollings, D. and Ritson, A. (1987) Immunocytochemical evidence that endometrial stromal granulocytes are granulated lymphocytes. *J. Pathol.*, **153**, 281–8.

Das, N. (1975) Advanced simultaneous intrauterine and abdominal pregnancy: a case report. *Br. J. Obstet. Gynaecol.*, **82**, 840–2.

Gibbs, R.S., O'Dell, I.N., MacGregor, R.R., Schwarz, R.H. and Morton, H. (1975) Puerperal endometritis: a prospective microbiologic study. *Am. J. Obstet. Gynecol.*, **121**, 919–25.

Honoré, L.H. and Nickerson, K.H. (1977) Combined intrauterine and tubal ectopic pregnancy: a possible case of superfetation. *Am. J. Obstet. Gynecol.*, **127**, 885–7.

Pijnenborg, R., Dixon, G., Robertson, W.B. and Brosens, I. (1980) Trophoblastic invasion of human decidua from 8 to 18 weeks of pregnancy. *Placenta*, **1**, 3–19.

Randall, S., Buckley, C.H. and Fox, H. (1987) Placentation in the Fallopian tube. *Int. J. Gynecol. Pathol.*, **6**, 132–9.

Robertson, W.B. (1981) *The Endometrium*, Butterworths, London.

Robertson, W.B., Khong, T.Y., Brosens, I., DeWolf, F., Sheppard, B.L. and Bonnar, J. (1986) Placental bed biopsy: a review from three European centres. *Am. J. Obstet. Gynecol.*, **155**, 401–12.

Rushton, D.I. (1987) Pathology of abortion. In *Haines and Taylor: Textbook of Obstetrical and Gynaecological Pathology* (ed. H. Fox), Churchill Livingstone, Edinburgh, pp. 1117–48.

Russell, P. (1987) Infections of the placental villi (villitis). In *Haines and Taylor: Textbook of Obstetrical and Gynaecological Pathology* (ed. H. Fox), Churchill Livingstone, Edinburgh, pp. 1014–29.

14   Gestational trophoblastic disease

The term 'gestational trophoblastic disease' encompasses hydatidiform moles, choriocarcinoma and placental site trophoblastic tumour, all of which are defined in strictly morphological terms (Table 14.1). A diagnosis of 'persistent trophoblastic disease' is made when plasma hCG levels remain elevated, or increase, after evacuation of a mole and this term does not, therefore, indicate or presuppose any specific histopathological findings. Many patients with persistent trophoblastic disease are treated, empirically but successfully, with chemotherapy without any attempt being made to establish a morphological diagnosis

Table 14.1 Histopathological classification of gestational trophoblastic disease

Complete hydatidiform mole
Partial hydatidiform mole
Invasive hydatidiform mole
Choriocarcinoma
Placental site trophoblastic tumour

and in this respect the role of the pathologist in the management of trophoblastic disease has been much diminished. Some women with persistent trophoblastic disease are, however, subjected to curettage and interpretation of these biopsies is notoriously difficult. Other problems posed to the pathologist are the distinction between partial moles, complete moles and hydropic abortions, the diagnosis of choriocarcinoma in women presenting with vaginal bleeding and the distinction between an exaggerated placental site reaction and a placental site trophoblastic tumour. These problems are at their most acute in curettage material and it is largely because of this that trophoblastic disease is considered in this volume.

248

14.1   Hydatidiform mole

Hydatidiform moles of all types are a form of abortion, and are not, as is often implied, benign neoplasms, the ability of molar tissue to invade and to metastasize to extrauterine sites being shared by normal placental trophoblast. It is only within recent years that a distinction has been drawn between complete and partial hydatidiform moles. Either form may progress to an invasive mole or to persistent trophoblastic disease (Mostoufi-Zadeh *et al.*, 1987) though this probably occurs more commonly with the complete mole.

14.1.1   Complete hydatidiform mole

About 90% of complete moles have a 46XX chromosomal constitution, the remainder being 46XY (Elston, 1987). In all cases the genome is of wholly paternal (androgenetic) origin and in the vast majority of XX moles there appears to be fertilization of an 'empty' ovum by a single haploid sperm which then duplicates without cytokinesis (Jacobs *et al.*, 1980), such moles being classed as monospermic or homozygous. All XY

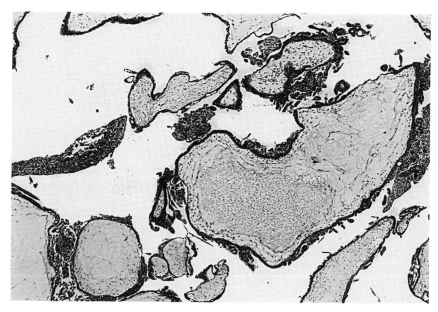

Figure 14.1   Complete hydatidiform mole. The villi are all abnormally large, show abnormal trophoblastic proliferation and lack fetal vessels. Haematoxylin and Eosin × 37.

moles and a small proportion of XX moles appear to be the result of fertilization of an 'empty' ovum by two haploid sperms which then fuse and replicate (Surti *et al.*, 1982), these being classed as dispermic or heterozygous moles. Interestingly, heterozygous moles are more likely to be complicated by persistent trophoblastic disease, and possibly choriocarcinoma, than are homozygous moles (Wake *et al.*, 1987).

In a complete hydatidiform mole a fetus is absent and there is generalized vesicular distension of the villi, the entire villous population being involved: the vesicular villi are usually evident to the naked eye in material retrieved by curettage but tend to be collapsed, and not grossly visible, in tissue obtained by suction. Histologically (Figure 14.1), the distension of the villi is seen to be due to an accumulation of fluid in the villous stroma and there is commonly central cavitation (cistern formation). The villi have a generally rounded contour and stromal vessels are usually absent, attenuated vestiges of such vessels being apparent in only a small minority of cases. All moles show, by definition, some degree of atypical trophoblastic proliferation, though this is not necessarily present in all the villi, some of which may have a flattened trophoblastic mantle. Most villi do, however, show trophoblastic proliferation, and this may be circumferential, focal or multifocal (Figures 14.2, 14,3) and of slight, moderate or marked degree (Figures 14.4, 14.5 and 14.6). It should be noted that as marked, or even greater, trophoblastic proliferation than that encountered in a mole may be seen in villi from a normal first trimester pregnancy: in the normal placenta, however, proliferating trophoblast is always at one pole, or along one side, of the villus (Figure 14.7) and never shows the focal or circumferential pattern characteristic of a mole. Variable nuclear atypia is invariably present in proliferating trophoblast though this is commonly no more marked than the atypia often seen in normal first trimester placentas.

Women who have had a complete hydatidiform mole have a small but definite risk of developing a subsequent choriocarcinoma and it has been suggested that the magnitude of this risk can be estimated by grading the degree of trophoblastic proliferation, the possibility of an eventual choriocarcinoma increasing progressively with the degree of tropho-blastic proliferation and atypia (Hertig and Sheldon, 1947). We do not grade complete hydatidiform moles and indeed would actively dissuade pathologists from attempting to grade these lesions. We take this attitude for the following reasons:

i. More recent studies have shown that the degree of trophoblastic proliferation is of little or no prognostic value (Elston, 1987).

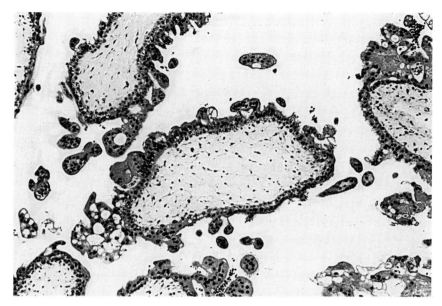

Figure 14.2 Complete hydatidiform mole. The central villus shows multifocal trophoblastic hyperplasia. Haematoxylin and Eosin × 117.

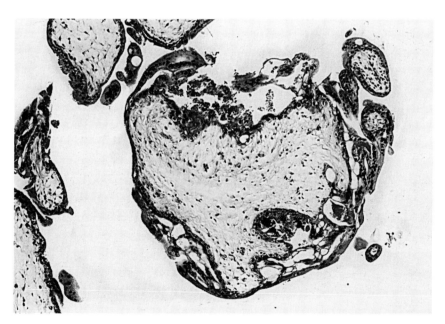

Figure 14.3 Complete hydatidiform mole. Circumferential trophoblastic hyperplasia. Haematoxylin and Eosin × 117.

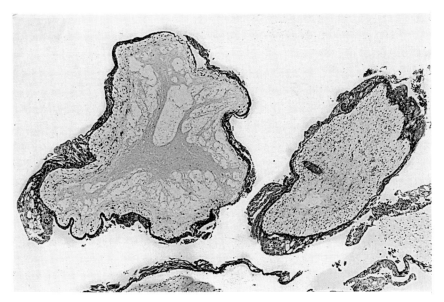

Figure 14.4 Complete hydatidiform mole showing a minor degree of trophoblastic proliferation. Haematoxylin and Eosin × 37.

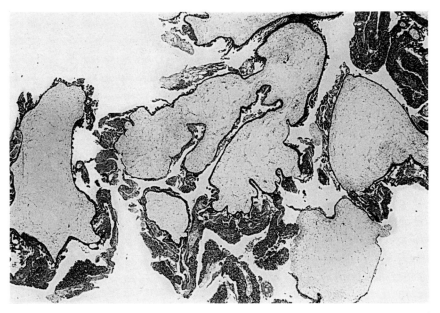

Figure 14.5 Complete hydatidiform mole showing a moderate degree of trophoblastic hyperplasia. Haematoxylin and Eosin × 37.

252

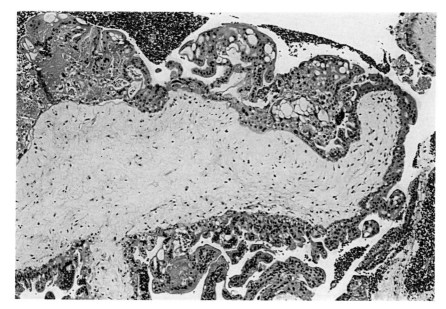

Figure 14.6 Complete hydatidiform mole showing a severe degree of circumferential trophoblastic hyperplasia. Haematoxylin and Eosin × 93.

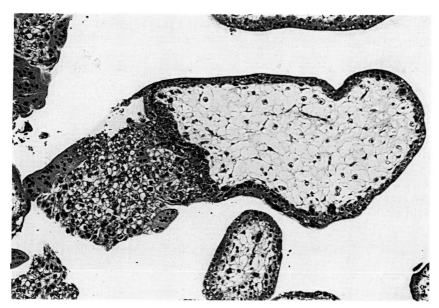

Figure 14.7 A normal first trimester placental villus showing the typical polar trophoblastic growth which is quite distinct from the circumferential or multifocal trophoblastic proliferation of molar pregnancy. Haematoxylin and Eosin × 149.

253

ii. The practice of prognostic grading may lead to the unjustified use of prophylactic chemotherapy in some patients and to unwarranted neglect of others.

iii. Grading has become obsolete since the introduction of radio-immunoassay for hCG; it is mandatory that all patients who have had a complete mole are followed up by serial hCG estimations, irrespective of the histological findings in the mole.

Because a diagnosis of a complete mole initiates a lengthy follow-up period it is important to ensure that curettage material from a hydropic abortion is not confused with a complete mole. In a hydropic abortus the distended villi rarely attain a size where they become macroscopically visible, only a proportion of the villi are hydropic (the others being generally fibrotic), central cavitation is not seen and, most importantly, the trophoblastic covering of the swollen villi is thin and attenuated, there being no evidence of atypical trophoblastic proliferation. Trophoblastic buds may persist in the hydropic villi but these are always at one edge or pole.

14.1.2   Partial hydatidiform mole

This term is applied to a mole in which only a small proportion of the villi show vesicular change associated with trophoblastic proliferation. The vast majority of partial hydatiform moles have a triploid karyotype, usually 69XXY but occasionally 69XXX or 69XYY (Lawler *et al.*, 1982); very occasional partial moles have been associated with a trisomy or a 46XX karyotype (Elston, 1987). Not all placentas from fetal triploidies take the form of a partial mole and it has been suggested that if the additional chromosomal load is of paternal origin a partial mole will result whilst if the extra chromosomal material is derived from the mother the gestation will be non-molar (Jacobs *et al.*, 1982).

In a partial hydatidiform mole a fetus is commonly present and hence fetal tissue may be seen in curetted material. Histologically, villi showing vesicular change are scattered amidst a villous population of normal size (Figure 14.8). Fetal vessels are often seen both in the villi of normal calibre and in the distended villi. The vesicular villi are rarely as large as are those seen in a complete mole, frequently show central cistern formation and, very characteristically, have an irregular, deeply indented outline (the 'Norwegian fjord' or 'coast of Ireland' appearance) (Figure 14.9). A degree of trophoblastic proliferation is always present in at least some of the vesicular villi though this is usually focal and rarely as marked as that seen in the complete mole (Figure 14.10).

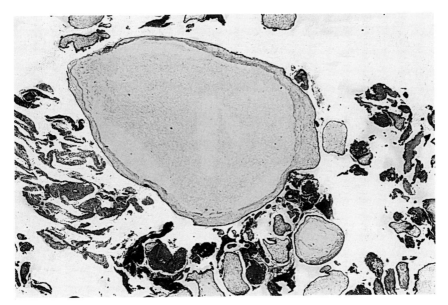

Figure 14.8 Partial hydatidiform mole. The field shows the typical mixture of small villi of normal configuration and a large vesicular villus. Haematoxylin and Eosin × 18.5.

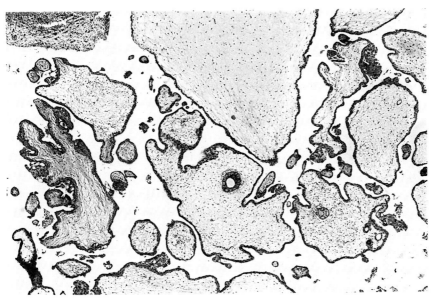

Figure 14.9 Partial hydatidiform mole showing the 'fjörd-like' irregular contour of the villi. Haematoxylin and Eosin × 37.

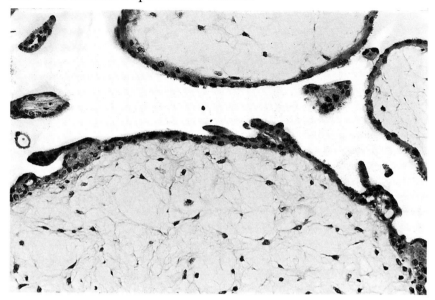

Figure 14.10 Partial hydatidiform mole showing the minimal trophoblastic hyperplasia seen in many such pregnancies. Haematoxylin and Eosin × 186.

The natural history of partial hydatidiform moles is still not fully defined though it is now clear that some can progress to an invasive mole and to persistent trophoblastic disease (Elston, 1987). It is therefore currently recommended that all patients with a partial hydatidiform mole are followed up by serial hCG estimations in exactly the same way as are those who have had a complete mole. The distinction in biopsy material between a partial and a complete hydatidiform mole is therefore of academic rather than practical importance, whilst that between a partial mole and a hydropic abortion assumes considerable significance. The criterion for making this distinction is the contrast between the highly irregular vesicular villi with central cistern formation and focal trophoblastic hyperplasia seen in the partial mole and the rounded villi, lacking cisternal change and showing no abnormal trophoblastic proliferation, in a hydropic abortion.

14.1.3   Invasive hydatidiform mole

An invasive mole is one in which vesicular villi invade the myometrium or its blood vessels: by implication, this term also applies to cases of extrauterine molar 'metastasis'.

Except under unusual circumstances, when curetted tissue contains fragments of myometrium invaded by molar villi, an invasive mole cannot be diagnosed in biopsy material. The mere presence in curettings of residual molar villi after evacuation of a mole does not justify a diagnosis of invasive mole; under these circumstances a comment should be made that the findings are compatible with persistent trophoblastic disease.

14.2   Choriocarcinoma

A choriocarcinoma may occur after a normal pregnancy, a spontaneous abortion or a hydatidiform mole, 50% of cases being preceded by a molar gestation. Classically, nodules of choriocarcinoma show extensive central necrosis with only a thin peripheral rim of viable tumour tissue, a feature reflecting the lack of an intrinsic tumour vasculature and one which results in curettage specimens from cases of choriocarcinoma often containing only necrotic tissue. Viable tumour has a characteristically bilaminar structure which recapitulates the appearance of the trophoblast

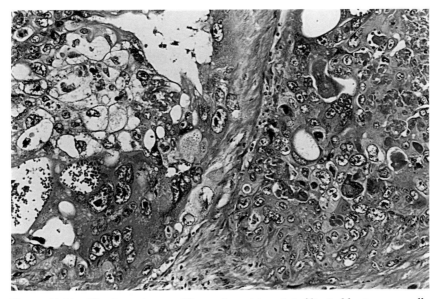

Figure 14.11   Choriocarcinoma. The endometrium is infiltrated by tumour cells which resemble syncytiotrophoblast to the lower left and cytotrophoblast to the upper left. Note the large, bizarre nuclei with prominent nucleoli and the absence of villous structures. Haemorrhage is often present. Haematoxylin and Eosin × 186.

of the implanting blastocyst (Figure 14.11), central cores of cytotropho-blastic cells being covered by rims or 'caps' of syncytiotrophoblast. Atypia and mitotic activity are seen but are often no more marked than is the case in the trophoblast of a normal blastocyst. Appearances such as these are rarely, if ever, seen in curettage material and the biopsy diagnosis of a choriocarcinoma presents considerable practical difficulties. Curettage to confirm a possible diagnosis of choriocarcinoma is usually undertaken when vaginal bleeding occurs following either a non-molar or a molar gestation and is still sometimes performed in patients with persistent trophoblastic disease. A logical approach to the interpretation of the findings in such curettings has been proposed by Elston (1987). If the curettings contain trophoblastic tissue this can be divided into three categories:

  i. Villous trophoblast.
 ii. Simple or suspicious non-villous trophoblast.
iii. Non-villous trophoblast diagnostic of choriocarcinoma.

The term 'villous trophoblast' indicates that placental villi, either of normal or molar type, are present in the curettings. The term 'simple non-

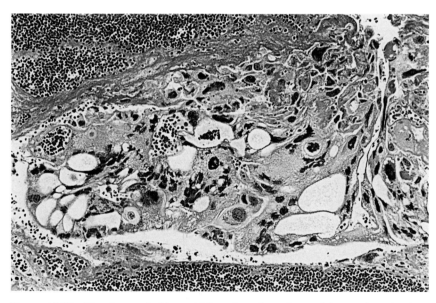

Figure 14.12 Simple trophoblast. Although at first glance this may be mistaken for choriocarcinoma, the trophoblast is not infiltrating but intimately mixed with blood and was seen in curettings that were carried out following persistent bleeding after a spontaneous abortion. Haematoxylin and Eosin × 370.

villous trophoblast' refers to small fragments of pyknotic trophoblastic cells with no clear distinction into cytotrophoblast and syncytiotrophoblast (Figure 14.12) whilst 'suspicious non-villous trophoblast' indicates the presence of trophoblastic tissue showing a bilaminar arrangement of cytotrophoblast and syncytiotrophoblast but without evidence of tissue invasion (Figure 14.13). The expression 'non-villous trophoblast diagnostic of choriocarcinoma' is only used when the curettings contain myometrial fragments that are being invaded by bilaminar trophoblast.

Interpretation of the significance of these findings depends upon a knowledge of the nature of the antecedent pregnancy. If the preceding pregnancy was a molar gestation the finding of villous trophoblast, simple non-villous trophoblast or suspicious non-villous trophoblast indicates a diagnosis of persistent trophoblastic disease and the patient will require continuing follow-up. If the previous gestation was a normal pregnancy or a spontaneous abortion the presence of villous trophoblast indicates retained products of conception. By contrast, the finding of non-villous trophoblast of either simple or suspicious type is an almost certain indication of choriocarcinoma and immediate full investigation should be instigated.

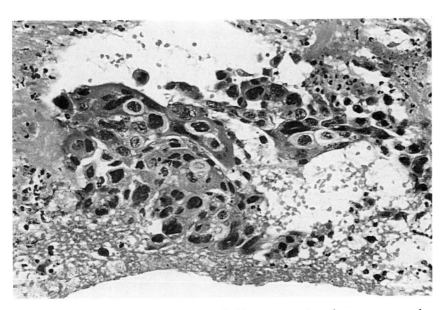

Figure 14.13 Suspicious persistent trophoblast in curettings from a woman who continued to bleed after aborting a hydatidiform mole. The sample contains fragments of proliferating syncytio- and cytotrophoblast mixed with fibrin. Tissue invasion is not seen. Haematoxylin and Eosin × 186.

Two points require stressing. A diagnosis of choriocarcinoma should *never* be made if villi are present in curettings and a pathologist *cannot* evaluate the significance of non-villous trophoblast in curettings without an adequate history which details the nature of the previous pregnancy.

14.3 Placental site trophoblastic tumour

Most neoplasms of this type follow a normal term pregnancy and whilst the clinical picture is very variable about 50% of patients present with amenorrhoea (Elston, 1987). This tumour is derived from the interstitial extravillous cytotrophoblastic cells of the placental bed; the lesion was originally regarded as an exaggerated placental site reaction or as a pseudotumour but is now recognized to be neoplastic (Young and Scully, 1984). A placental site trophoblastic tumour forms a mass involving the endometrium and myometrium and is composed predominantly of mononuclear cytotrophoblastic-like cells which infiltrate between and dissect the myometrial fibres (Figure 14.14) as cords or sheets. Necrosis and haemorrhage are often noticeably absent. Though the classical bimorphic pattern of a choriocarcinoma is not seen a number of

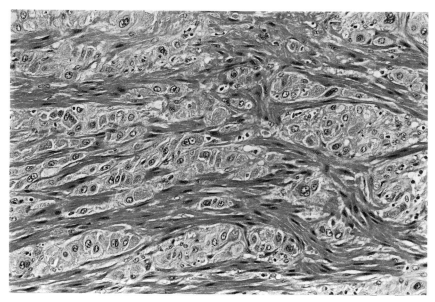

Figure 14.14 Placental site trophoblastic tumour. The cytotrophoblastic cells are of bland appearance and are infiltrating the myometrium without necrosis or haemorrhage. Haematoxylin and Eosin × 186.

irregularly distributed multinucleate cells are usually present. The cytotrophoblastic-like cells that predominate in these neoplasms tend to stain positively for hPL rather than hCG (Kurman *et al.*, 1984). The endometrium adjacent to the neoplastic cells may have a pseudodecidual change and entrapped vessels not uncommonly show fibrinoid necrosis. Most placental site trophoblastic tumours appear to be benign but between 10 and 15% behave in a malignant fashion (Young *et al.*, 1988).

The diagnosis of a placental site trophoblastic tumour in curettings is far from easy, the major difficulty being in attempting to distinguish between a neoplasm of this type and an exaggerated, but non-neoplastic, placental site reaction. One of the most useful criteria in making this differential diagnosis is the clinical history, for the longer the time interval between the previous pregnancy and curettings the more likely is it that infiltrating cytotrophoblastic cells are neoplastic in nature. Findings suggestive of an exaggerated placental site reaction include the presence of true decidua and placental villi, the presence of a relatively large number of multinucleated trophoblastic cells and an absence of mitotic figures. By contrast, features indicating a diagnosis of placental site trophoblastic tumour are the presence of sheets or confluent masses of cytotrophoblastic cells, a paucity of multinucleated cells and the presence of mitotic figures. To complicate still further the distinction between a placental site trophoblastic tumour and an exaggerated placental site reaction it has recently been recognized that the normal trophoblast of the placental site can assume an aggregated pattern to form a 'placental site nodule' (Young *et al.*, 1988). These nodules, usually single but occasionally multiple, are well circumscribed, oval, elongated or rounded and are typically eosinophilic and prominently hyalinized. Placental site nodules can be distinguished from a true placental site trophoblastic tumour by their circumscribed, non-infiltrative nature, their lack of mitotic activity and their tendency to undergo hyalinization.

The distinction between a placental site tumour and a choriocarcinoma in curettings can also prove difficult but a preponderance of cytotrophoblast, a relative or absolute absence of syncytiotrophoblast, a haphazard juxtaposition of cytotrophoblast and any multinucleated cells that may be present and a lack of haemorrhage and necrosis all point to a diagnosis of placental site trophoblastic turmour. In equivocal cases staining for hPL and hCG may help to resolve the dilemma, the true choriocarcinoma showing extensive positive staining for hCG and the placental site tumour tending to stain predominantly for hPL.

Assessment of the degree of malignancy of a placental site trophoblastic tumour is difficult, largely because criteria for distinguishing benign from malignant placental site trophoblastic tumours have not yet been firmly established. It has been claimed that tumours with a mitotic count of less than 2 per 10 high power fields behave in a benign fashion (Young and Scully, 1984) but nevertheless one neoplasm with only 2 mitotic figures per 10 high power fields pursued a highly malignant course and proved fatal (Eckstein *et al.*, 1982). There is little doubt that a placental site trophoblastic tumour with a high mitotic count should be considered as being at least potentially malignant but a false sense of security should not be engendered by a low mitotic count. Whether or not the degree of atypia in the neoplasm is of prognostic importance is currently undecided.

References

Eckstein, R.P., Paradinas, F.J. and Bagshawe, K.D. (1982) Placental site trophoblastic tumour (trophoblastic pseudotumour): a study of four cases requiring hysterectomy including one fatal case. *Histopathology*, **6**, 221–6.

Elston, C.W. (1987) Gestational trophoblastic disease. In *Haines and Taylor: Textbook of Obstetrical and Gynaecological Pathology* (ed. H. Fox), Churchill Livingstone, Edinburgh, pp. 1045–78.

Hertig, A.T. and Sheldon, W.H. (1947) Hydatidiform mole: a pathologico-clinical correlation of 200 cases. *Am. J. Obstet. Gynecol.*, **53**, 1–36.

Jacobs, P.A., Szulman, A.E., Funkmouska, J., Maatsura, J.S. and Wilson, C.C. (1982) Human triploidy: relationship between parental origin of the additional haploid complement and development of partial hydatidiform mole. *Ann. Hum. Genetics*, **46**, 223–31.

Jacobs, P.A., Wilson, C.M., Sprenkle, J.A., Rosenhein, N.B. and Migeon, B.R. (1980) Mechanism of origin of complete hydatidiform moles. *Nature*, **286**, 714–16.

Kurman, R.J., Young, R.H., Norris, H.J., Lawrence, W.D. and Scully, R.E. (1984) Immunocytochemical localization of placental lactogen and chorionic gonadotrophin in the normal placenta and trophoblastic tumors with emphasis on intermediate trophoblast and the placental site trophoblastic tumor. *Int. J. Gynecol. Pathol.*, **3**, 101–21.

Lawler, S.D., Fisher, R.A., Pickhall, V.J., Povey, S. and Evans, M.W. (1982) Genetic studies on hydatidiform moles. I. The origin of partial moles. *Cancer, Genetics. Cytogen.*, **5**, 309–20.

Mostoufi-Zadeh, M., Berkowitz, R.S. and Driscoll, S.G. (1987) Persistence of partial mole. *Am. J. Clin. Pathol.*, **87**, 377–80.

Surti, U., Szulman, A.E. and O'Brien, S. (1982) Dispermic origin and clinical outcome of three complete hydatidiform moles with 46XY karotype. *Am. J. Obstet. Gynecol.*, **144**, 84–7.

Wake, N., Fujino, T., Hoshi, S., Shinkai, N., Sakai, K., Kato, H., Hashimoto, M., Uasuda, T., Yamada, H. and Ichinoe, K. (1987) The propensity to malignancy of dispermic heterozygous moles. *Placenta*, **8**, 319–26.

Young, R.H. and Scully, R.E. (1984) Placental site trophoblastic tumor: current status. *Clin. Obstet. Gynecol.*, **27**, 248–58.

Young, R.H., Kurman, R.J. and Scully, R.E. (1988) Proliferations and tumors of the placental site. *Semin. Diagn. Pathol.*, **5**, 223–37.

15 Endometrial biopsy in specific circumstances

In the preceding chapters of this book endometrial biopsies have been discussed in terms of specific pathological lesions of the endometrium, such as inflammation, hyperplasia or neoplasia. In daily practice, however, most endometrial biopsies received in the laboratory are accompanied by clinical information which is couched in terms of the patient's symptoms rather than in terms of a suggested pathological lesion. Thus the request form usually specifies complaints, for example 'infertility' or 'postmenopausal bleeding', without suggesting a specific diagnosis, such as chronic endometritis or endometrial adenocarcinoma. It may also describe problems that have occurred during the procedure (Figure 15.1). In this chapter therefore we consider the approach to endometrial biopsies in women with particular symptoms, acknowledging that we are, to a considerable extent, reiterating information already remarked upon in relationship to specific pathological processes.

During the reproductive years of a woman's life the most common indications for endometrial biopsy are abnormal uterine bleeding and infertility. Curettage is also performed frequently for complications of pregnancy, sometimes for diagnostic purposes but often for therapeutic reasons. In the peri- and postmenopausal years the principal indication for biopsy is abnormal uterine bleeding whilst not uncommonly curettage is undertaken to exclude an endometrial abnormality in women being treated for unrelated gynaecological disorders, such as uterine prolapse.

15.1 Abnormal bleeding during the reproductive years

Uterine bleeding may be abnormal in respect to its frequency, duration, quantity or the age at which it occurs and may take several clinical forms (Table 15.1). Although the menstrual disturbance cannot always be exactly correlated with the underlying pathological process, the clinical features will often supply a clue to the possible nature of the abnormality. In practice, the pathologist should be aware that a term such as

263

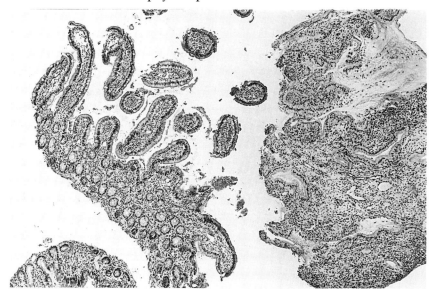

Figure 15.1 Small intestinal mucosa and endocervical tissue in an endometrial biopsy. The surgeon thought that uterine perforation had occurred during the procedure. Haematoxylin and Eosin × 60.

menorrhagia may be used on a histopathological request form in a rather general manner to refer to any type of abnormal or excessive bleeding. Care has also to be taken to distinguish between single episodes of heavy bleeding, which may be the result, for example, of recent pregnancy and those episodes which persist or recur and for which a potentially more serious underlying cause should be sought.

Table 15.1 Terminology of clinical symptoms

Amenorrhoea	the absence of menstruation, primary and secondary
Oligomenorrhoea	infrequent menstruation
Hypomenorrhoea	scanty menstruation
Menorrhagia	regular cyclical bleeding which is heavy or prolonged
Polymenorrhoea	cyclical bleeding which occurs more frequently than usual but is not abnormally heavy
Polymenorrhagia or menometrorrhagia	frequent episodes of heavy bleeding
Metrorrhagia	continuous or intermittent irregular, non-cyclical bleeding, including postmenopausal and intermenstrual bleeding

(After Tindall, 1987.)

15.1.1   *Amenorrhoea*

(a) *Primary amenorrhoea* rarely necessitates biopsy of the endometrium, investigations being largely concerned with the identification of a genital tract, chromosomal or endocrinological abnormality. In those rare cases in which biopsy is undertaken, we have seen both inactive, atrophic endometrium (Figure 3.22) and inactive endometrium with a shallow, rather poorly developed functionalis, the appearances depending upon the degree of oestrogenic deprivation (Figure 3.24).

(b) *Secondary amenorrhoea*, that is amenorrhoea preceded by spontaneous menstruation, may be the result of conditions which are physiological, such as those that often occur in the postmenarchal, but still adolescent, girl, pregnancy (which surprisingly is not always suspected by the patient) lactation and the menopause, or those which occur at inappropriate times and are the consequence of a pathological process.

The latter occur in patients with developing or established ovarian failure due to a variety of causes (severe systemic illness, lesions in the

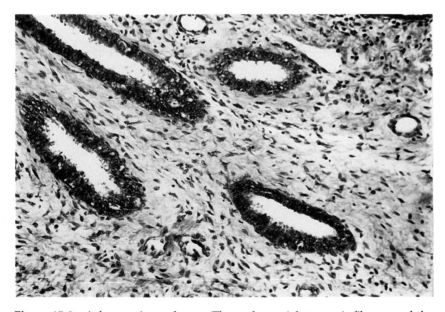

Figure 15.2 Asherman's syndrome. The endometrial stroma is fibrous and the glands narrow and inactive. At subsequent hysterectomy more normal proliferative endometrium was identified elsewhere in the uterine cavity. Haematoxylin and Eosin × 186.

cerebral cortex, hypothalamus, pituitary or ovary) or, less commonly, are due to abnormalities in the uterus itself. This symptom is therefore common to women with a wide variety of clinical disorders but, when the amenorrhoea is the consequence of ovarian failure, the appearances of the endometrium are similar whatever the underlying abnormality; the endometrial biopsy resembles that seen in the postmenopausal woman (Chapters 2 and 3).

Very rarely, secondary amenorrhoea, or, more commonly, oligomenorrhoea, is the consequence of endometrial damage due to tuberculosis, radiation (although amenorrhoea in these circumstances is usually secondary to ovarian failure) or Asherman's syndrome. The latter, also known as intrauterine synechiae, fibrotic endometritis or traumatic hypomenorrhoea-amenorrhoea, is characterized by the presence of adhesions between the surfaces of the uterine cavity which are usually a consequence of post-abortive curettage, particularly in the presence of sepsis. They may also, rarely, follow myomectomy or Caesarean section. The uterine curettings in Asherman's syndrome are typically scanty and composed of endometrium completely or partly lacking evidence of normal cyclical changes, with fibrosed, or even ossified, scarred stroma and sparse, inactive glands which may be cystically dilated (Figure 15.2).

15.1.2   Scanty bleeding

(a)   *Hypomenorrhoea*   This is, by definition, the occurrence of menstrual periods which last less than two days. The cause is nearly always constitutional and in these cases the endometrial biopsy will almost certainly be normal in appearance for the stated day of the cycle. In some patients, however, scanty periods may presage the onset of amenorrhoea and in that case the abnormalities described above may be seen.

(b)   *Oligomenorrhoea*   Infrequent, and often irregular, periods may, rarely, occur in women who are normally fertile but are more commonly encountered in patients with an ovulatory defect and this symptom is therefore of more significance than simple hypomenorrhoea.

In the patient with constitutional oligomenorrhoea, the variations in cycle length appear to be due entirely to prolongation or arrest of the preovulatory phase, the secretory phase remaining remarkably constant at 14 days. The appearance of the endometrium will vary, therefore, according to the stage in the cycle at which the biopsy has been taken. During the follicular phase a picture of weak or normal proliferative activity or, in some cases, of prolonged proliferation is seen and maturation will appear to be retarded if related only to the date of the last menstrual period. Once ovulation has occurred the appearance of the secretory endometrium is consistent with the date of ovulation unless, however, the patient also has a luteal phase insufficiency.

More significantly, infrequent menstruation may also be indicative of developing ovarian failure or of the polycystic ovary syndrome and the appearance of the endometrium under these circumstances is very variable. The endometrial pattern may range from the inactive, post-menopausal type picture associated with low oestrogen production seen in patients with ovarian failure through varying degrees of hyperplasia in women with the polycystic ovary syndrome who have a hyper-oestrogenic state associated with non-ovulatory follicular development, to an endometrium of normal appearance if, by chance, the patient has recently had a normal cycle.

15.1.3   Excessive bleeding

In this text, we are concerned only with those abnormalities of bleeding that originate within the uterine body and not those which arise in the tubes, lower genital tract or cervix, or are the result of abnormalities of haemostasis. It should be mentioned, however, that defects in local haemostatic mechanism are a common and important cause of excessive bleeding from a morphologically normal uterus (Sheppard, 1984). The single most common cause of abnormal uterine bleeding during the reproductive years is pregnancy or, more precisely, abnormalities of pregnancy, in particular threatened or inevitable abortion or ectopic gestation.

In many other patients, however, examination of the endometrium reveals no abnormality, because the cause of the abnormal bleeding lies elsewhere. There may be abnormalities outside the uterus, e.g. pelvic infection or endometriosis, or within the myometrium or vasculature of the uterus. There may be defects in haemostatic mechanisms, endocrine abnormalities or psychiatric disorders. The bleeding may also have its origin in the vagina or cervix and thus not be abnormal uterine bleeding in the strict meaning of the word.

In those women in whom an endometrial abnormality is observed, the fault in some lies in the hypothalamic-pituitary-ovarian axis, the endometrial changes reflecting abnormalities of ovarian hormone secretion, whilst in others there may be an intrinsic endometrial lesion.

(a)   *Menorrhagia*   Unduly heavy periods occur most frequently when there is an increase in the surface area of the endometrium, e.g. in patients with submucous leiomyomas, adenomyosis, uterine polyps (Figure 8.13) or uterus didelphis or bicornis. In such cases the endometrium may be entirely normal or there may be thinning of the endometrium where it overlies a leiomyoma (Figure 1.6) or where it is ulcerated and/or inflamed at the tip of a polypoidal submucous leiomyoma. In patients with uterus bicornis, it is important to recognize that the samples obtained from the two halves of the uterus may not be identical, e.g. there may be a pregnancy in one horn whilst curettings from the second horn may strongly suggest the possibility of an ectopic gestation.

Menorrhagia occurs in a proportion of IUCD users and endometrial biopsy in such cases may reveal the full range of histological features described in Chapter 6; this symptom may also be indicative of luteal phase insufficiency (Chapter 4) but this condition more commonly causes occasional heavy periods rather than persistent menorrhagia.

When menorrhagia is due to faults in the haemostatic mechanisms there may be no morphological abnormality but it must be remembered that bleeding can be a consequence of a neoplastic process in the haemopoietic tissues; thus there may be, for example, a leukaemic infiltrate of the endometrium. In patients with congestive cardiac failure

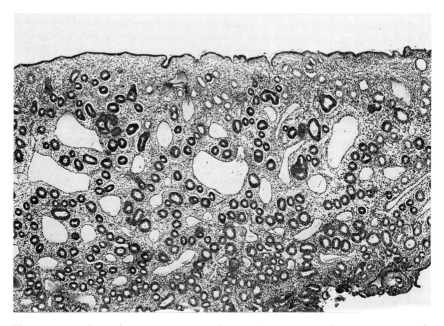

Figure 15.3 Lymphangiectasia in the endometrium of a woman with menorrhagia. The significance of this finding was never satisfactorily explained but may have been a complication of the leiomyomas which were present in the uterus. Haematoxylin and Eosin × 37.

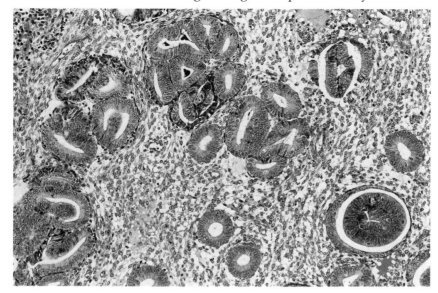

Figure 15.4 The endometrium in a patient with menorrhagia. Apparent crowding of the glands in this example was thought to be due to traumatic loss of stroma occurring during curettage. Note also the 'gland-within-gland' appearance at the lower right; this too is an artifact. Haematoxylin and Eosin × 149.

haemorrhagic infarction of the endometrium (uterine apoplexy) may result in heavy vaginal bleeding (Daly and Balogh, 1968).

Occasionally, an endometrial biopsy in women with menorrhagia reveals an abnormality the significance of which may be difficult to evaluate. Two of these are illustrated in Figures 15.3 and 15.4.

(b) *Polymenorrhoea* Regular periods, but occurring more frequently than every 22 days, are due to a short follicular phase and are the consequence either of disturbances in the hypothalamic-pituitary-ovarian axis or of alterations in ovarian function consequent upon pelvic infection or endometriosis; polymenorrhoea may occur for a short time when ovulation returns following pregnancy.

The appearances of the endometrium are usually normal in relation to the date of ovulation but appear accelerated if related only to the date of the last menstrual period.

(c) *Polymenorrhagia* This is a combination of frequent and heavy bleeding which is usually the consequence of uterine or ovarian dysfunction, being seen particularly in patients with pelvic infection. There may be no abnormality in the endometrial biopsy or there may be an inflammatory cell infiltrate composed predominantly of haemosiderin-laden macrophages with scanty plasma cells and lymphocytes (Figure 7.3). It is a debatable point whether the inflammation is the cause of the excess bleeding or is its consequence. The sparse nature of the inflammation in most cases and the absence of any disturbance in the hormonal response suggest that in most instances it is the result of the repeated tissue breakdown rather than its cause.

(d) *Metrorrhagia* This is continuous or intermittent non-cyclical bleeding and includes intermenstrual and postmenopausal bleeding. Metrorrhagia has a wide variety of causes varying from disturbances of ovarian function, such as anovulatory cycles or luteal phase insufficiency, to intrauterine neoplasms or the demise of an intrauterine or ectopic gestation. Whilst careful timing of the biopsy is usually recommended when evaluating the endometrium in infertile patients, biopsy as soon as possible is more appropriate in patients with metrorrhagia as there is nothing to gain by delaying the procedure and, indeed, further loss of tissue may hamper diagnosis.

The appearance of the endometrium in patients having anovulatory cycles is very variable. The sample may be scanty, particularly if bleeding has been prolonged, and show little or no proliferative activity in a poorly formed shallow functionalis with evidence of stromal crumbling and interstitial haemorrhage. This is typical of the perimenopausal anovulatory state with low, or fluctuating, oestrogen levels in which oestrogen secretion has been sufficient to stimulate the endometrium and permit oestrogen withdrawal bleeding but has been insufficient for the development of a normal functionalis.

In the woman with polycystic ovary syndrome, or in the perimenarchal or perimenopausal woman in whom there is follicular development without ovulation, it is more usual to find a degree of simple hyperplasia but sometimes an atypical hyperplasia or even a carcinoma is encountered (Chapter 9). The history is typically that of a period of amenorrhoea followed by spotting which terminates in a heavy prolonged bleed, so-called metropathia haemorrhagica. A similar range of endometrial appearances is seen in the patient with an oestrogen-secreting ovarian neoplasm and in women who have been given unopposed oestrogen therapy at the menopause (Chapter 5). In those women in whom there is evidence of hyperplasia, progestagen therapy or induction of ovulation will, in the majority of cases, produce a reversion to normal. There is a small group of patients, however, in whom atypical hyperplasia persists despite progestagen therapy (Figure 5.14). Some of these women may eventually come to hysterectomy as a consequence of their failure to respond to a progestagen whilst, in a very small number, carcinoma may supervene. Youth is no guarantee of safety from the development of carcinoma and whilst neoplasia is not common in the premenopausal woman the possibility should always be borne in mind.

Intermenstrual bleeding often has a cause outside the uterine cavity, such as carcinoma of the cervix; fragments of such a neoplasm are sometimes found in curettings (Figure 15.5). This symptom may also have less sinister causes amongst which are ovulation bleeding, when the endometrial biopsy is normal, luteal phase insufficiency, characteristically presenting as premenstrual spotting (Chapter 4), the presence of endometrial or isthmic polyps and, in some women, the use of steroid contraceptives, although in the latter case the bleeding is not so much intermenstrual as inter-hormone withdrawal bleeding; the endometrial biopsy appearances in such cases are described in Chapter 5.

Both premenstrual spotting and prolonged periods are characteristic of luteal phase insufficiency, the former being due to the premature demise of the corpus luteum and a partial breakdown of the endometrium prior to the onset of menstruation and the latter to prolonged shedding of the endometrium (Chapter 4).

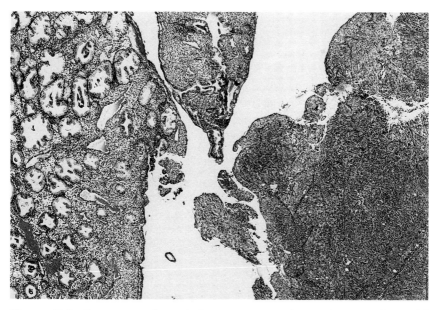

Figure 15.5 Fragments of cervical squamous carcinoma in an endometrial curetting. To the left there is normal secretory endometrium and to the right, non-keratinizing, large cell squamous carcinoma. Haematoxylin and Eosin × 93.

The appearances of the endometrial biopsy in abortions and in ectopic pregnancy are discussed in Chapter 13 and endometrial neoplasms, stromal, epithelial or mixed, which, rarely, may be associated with abnormal bleeding in the reproductive years are fully covered in Chapters 10 and 11.

15.2 Abnormal perimenopausal or postmenopausal bleeding

At the menopause, prior to the complete cessation of menstruation, the majority of women experience a gradual reduction in the amount and frequency of menstruation over a period of months or, less commonly, years. Less frequently, but equally normally, there may be an abrupt cessation of menstrual loss without prior warning. Biopsy of the endometrium is rarely carried out in these women, but when it is the appearances are generally unremarkable and vary according to the patient's hormonal status at the time of biopsy.

In contrast, heavy perimenstrual bleeding is never normal and women experiencing excessive bleeding frequently undergo biopsy.

15.2.1 *Perimenopausal bleeding*

The appearances of the endometrium vary greatly. Many of the more important features are described in the earlier section of this chapter dealing with the various forms of excessive bleeding. These will only be summarized here.

A shallow, poorly-developed, weakly-proliferative or inactive endometrium is characteristic of the patient with diminishing ovarian function and low oestrogen levels. Biopsy specimens from such patients are often technically unsatisfactory because they are so small and fragmented, and it may be possible to do no more than exclude the presence of a neoplasm in the material supplied. In such biopsies there is often evidence of spontaneous stromal crumbling, breakdown and interstitial haemorrhage together with weak proliferative activity and the assumption is often made that oestrogenic stimulation has been insufficient to maintain endometrial growth.

Simple endometrial hyperplasia is characteristic of the patient with ovulatory failure in whom there is follicular development but not follicular maturation, the resulting failure of progesterone secretion allowing for unopposed oestrogenic activity. Curettings in these cases are usually voluminous and it is important to exclude the presence of neoplasia or atypical hyperplasia.

Irregular shedding due to abnormal persistence of the corpus luteum is responsible for some cases of perimenopausal bleeding and other facets of luteal phase insufficiency are not uncommon, the features being as described on p. 53–66.

Endometrial adenocarcinoma is not common before the menopause but does occur and should always be suspected in women with perimenopausal or postmenopausal bleeding. Indeed, the presence of a carcinoma may well mask the development of the menopause as menstrual bleeding is replaced by bleeding due to the neoplasm. Stromal sarcomas, though less common than carcinomas, are more likely to occur in younger women and may therefore be identified not only in the perimenopausal patient but also in the woman of reproductive age.

Simple polyps and adenomyomatous polyps are commonly encountered and the pathologist should always be aware also of the possibility that the bleeding may have its origin in a cervical neoplasm. Great care should be taken to examine any cervical fragments included in the curettings (Figure 15.5).

15.2.2   Postmenopausal bleeding

Postmenopausal bleeding should always be regarded as due to the presence of a neoplasm until otherwise proven. Most commonly the tumour is an endometrial adenocarcinoma, these being fully described in Chapter 10. Postmenopausal bleeding may also occur in patients with metastatic carcinoma of the endometrium and the finding of multifocal tumour or a carcinoma of unusual morphology should always raise the possibility in the mind of the pathologist. A metastatic tumour is likely to have had a primary origin in the breast, ovary or large intestine (Figures 12.6 and 12.7).

In many women with postmenopausal bleeding curettings reveal an inactive endometrium showing no proliferative activity but with glandular epithelial stratification, a finding suggesting persistent, though very low, oestrogenic stimulation. In the early months or years of the postmenopausal state, a proliferative endometrium of unremarkable appearance is seen, such a finding, of course, becoming progressively less common as the time interval from the menopause increases.

Even long after the menopause, the endometrium retains the capacity to respond to oestrogenic stimulation and therefore if oestrogen is present a proliferative or hyperplastic picture may be induced. This occurs in women using topical vaginal or vulval oestrogen creams or receiving unopposed oestrogen replacement therapy, in a small proportion of women receiving Tamoxifen therapy for the treatment of breast carcinoma and in patients with an oestrogen-secreting ovarian neoplasm or a luteinized follicular cyst. This latter abnormality has been described as occurring up to seven years after the menopause.

Frequently, women presenting with postmenopausal bleeding have been given progestagen therapy before the endometrial biopsy is carried out and, if the oestrogen has induced progesterone receptors, stromal pseudodecidualization and glandular secretion may be apparent.

In some patients with typical senile, cystic atrophy the cystic tissue becomes polypoidal and removal of such polyps is usually followed by cessation of bleeding despite the absence of histological evidence of tissue breakdown in the polyp (Figure 15.6).

Postmenopausal bleeding or blood-stained discharge may also occur in women with endometrial inflammation (Chapter 7). This is usually non-specific and may be associated with a pyometra or, rarely, a utero-colonic fistula complicating diverticular disease of the large bowel. The endometrial biopsy may contain acute purulent material, non-specific granulation tissue, atrophic endometrium heavily infiltrated by histiocytes and lymphocytes together with metaplastic squamous epithelium in which there may, or may not, be cytological atypia. Postmenopausal bleeding may also complicate tuberculosis (p. 119) or malakoplakia (p. 117) and in both cases the curettings usually permit a specific diagnosis.

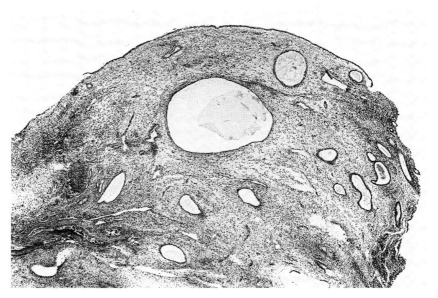

Figure 15.6 A polyp from a woman with postmenopausal bleeding. It is composed of inactive, rather atrophic endometrium in which many of the glands are cystically dilated. This is the appearance of senile cystic atrophy. Haematoxylin and Eosin × 37.

Thus endometrial biopsies from women with postmenopausal bleeding may reveal an adenocarcinoma, show evidence of continuing oestrogenic stimulation, indicate an inflammatory process or demonstrate polypoidal senile cystic change. The fact remains, however, that in a proportion of women complaining of postmenopausal bleeding the findings in the endometrial biopsy will reveal no morphological basis for this symptom.

15.3   Endometrial biopsy in the infertile patient

Endometrial biopsy specimens from infertile women are often rather small, having been taken with the intention of causing as little damage or disturbance to the endometrium as possible. They therefore require more than usual care in their handling, orientation and interpretation.

Endometrial biopsy, with accurate dating of the endometrium, is still regarded as an important component of the investigation of infertility (Annos et al., 1980; Rosenfeld et al., 1980) and interpretation of such biopsies depends heavily upon both close co-operation between the clinician and the pathologist and the receipt of accurate clinical information. It is important that, whenever possible, the appearances of the endometrium should be related to the date of ovulation and not to the date of the last menstrual period, this because of the variation in the length of the follicular phase. When the date of ovulation is not known with accuracy, there are two alternatives: the date on which mittelschmerz occurred may be ascertained or the usual cycle length and duration of the menstrual period may be used as a basis for estimating the probable date of ovulation.

In the majority of infertile women the morphology of the endometrial biopsy is normal and the appearances are approximately appropriate for the day of the cycle. This is the case when, as so often happens, the cause of the infertility lies outside the uterus, e.g. in women with the unruptured follicle syndrome in whom the pattern of hormonal secretion is normal but in whom the failure of ovum release precludes fertilization. In other cases, however, biopsy reveals an abnormality which may be due to a primary endometrial disorder or may be secondary to ovarian dysfunction. Generally speaking infertility due to ovarian dysfunction is often associated with menstrual disturbances or amenorrhoea whilst endometrial abnormalities are commonly unsuspected clinically.

15.3.1   Endometrial abnormalities

(a) *Inflammation.* Acute endometrial inflammation is not usually regarded as a cause of infertility but nevertheless may be indicative of infection elsewhere in the genital tract which may be the basis of infertility, for example in the cervix or Fallopian tubes. On the other hand, both non-specific and specific chronic endometritis are well recognized as a cause of infertility and also, in certain circumstances, of recurrent abortion.

In interpreting inflammation in the biopsy from an infertile patient care should be taken to distinguish between a focal inflammatory process, such as that seen on the surface of a polyp or submucous leiomyoma, where the inflammation may be irrelevant in relation to the infertility, and inflammation which affects the entire endometrium and is more likely to be of significance. Although leiomyomas are present in 3 to 5% of infertile women they are rarely submucous or apparent on endometrial biopsy; the relationship between infertility and their presence is uncertain.

Endometrial tuberculosis is now rarely seen in the United Kingdom but its association with infertility is well recognized. It is, however, the accompanying tubal disease which is the cause of the infertility and not the endometrial disease which is usually superficial, transient and rarely well established (Chapter 7). Clearly, any woman who is so ill with tuberculosis that she becomes amenorrhoeic will be infertile and endometrial disease will, in the absence of regular shedding, show evidence of caseation.

Even in the absence of active inflammation, post-inflammatory fibrosis, particularly that seen in Asherman's syndrome, may cause infertility. The biopsy appearances are discussed on p. 266.

In a small proportion of women with longstanding primary or secondary infertility there may be no evidence of active endometrial inflammation, the cyclical changes are appropriate for the hormonal status, secretory transformation is uniform and adequate, and microbiological cultures are negative but many of the glands contain epithelial cells and macrophages in the absence of any other evidence of inflammation (Figure 15.7). The aetiology and significance of this condition is unknown to us but this is a recurrent finding in patients with unexplained infertility.

15.3.2 Ovarian dysfunction

In infertile patients with oligomenorrhoea or amenorrhoea the endometrium may be shallow, poorly grown and either lacking in mitotic activity or exhibiting only weak proliferative activity, the appearances suggesting anovulation with low oestrogen levels. Alternatively there may be endometrial hyperplasia, suggesting anovulation with elevated or persistent oestrogen secretion. The latter is more likely to be associated with infrequent heavy bleeds interspersed with irregular spotting.

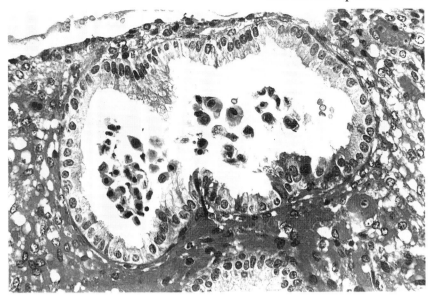

Figure 15.7   Endometrial biopsy from a patient with unexplained infertility. The secretory gland contains a cluster of histiocytes and epithelial cells. There is no evidence of active inflammation and secretory changes are uniform and adequate. Haematoxylin and Eosin × 370.

In some women, despite the presence of ovarian dysfunction, there may be little or no menstrual disturbance. Ovulation may occur but the patient may have a short luteal phase, and hence frequent menstruation. Luteal phase insufficiency may be unsuspected until the biopsy reveals evidence of a secretory abnormality (the features of which are described in Chapter 4). It should not be assumed that the infertility is necessarily the consequence of luteal phase insufficiency for the abnormality would have to be present in most cycles before it could be regarded as having any clinical significance. Care should also be exercised to prevent overdiagnosis of luteal phase abnormalities, particularly in the rather superficial biopsy typically received from the infertile patient. In the late secretory phase, when a well-developed superficial compact layer has formed, the glands in this part of the endometrium are often rather narrow and, to the unwary, they may misleadingly suggest a secretory defect (Figure 3.17).

Rarely, ovarian hormone production is normal but the endometrium fails to show the appropriate cyclical changes because of an insensitivity to the hormones (p. 66).

References

Annos, T., Thompson, I.E. and Taylor, M.L. (1980) Luteal phase deficiency and infertility: difficulties encountered in diagnosis and treatment. *Obstet. Gynecol.*, **55**, 705–10.

Daly, J.J. and Balogh, K., Jr (1968) Hemorrhagic necrosis of the senile endometrium ('apoplexia uteri'): relation to superficial hemorrhagic necrosis of the bowel. *New Engl. J. Med.*, **278**, 709–11.

Rosenfeld, D.L., Chodow, S. and Bronson, R.A. (1980) Diagnosis of luteal phase inadequacy. *Obstet. Gynecol.*, **56**, 193–6.

Sheppard, B.L. (1984) The pathology of dysfunctional uterine bleeding. *Clinics Obstet. Gynaecol.*, **11**, 227–36.

Tinall, V.R. (1987) Jeffcoate's Principles of Gynaecology, Butterworths, London, pp. 512.

Index

Page numbers in *italics* refer to figures, page numbers in **bold** refer to main entries.